STRENGTH AND CONDITIONING FOR CYCLISTS

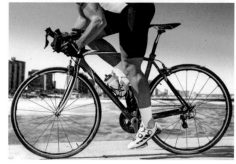

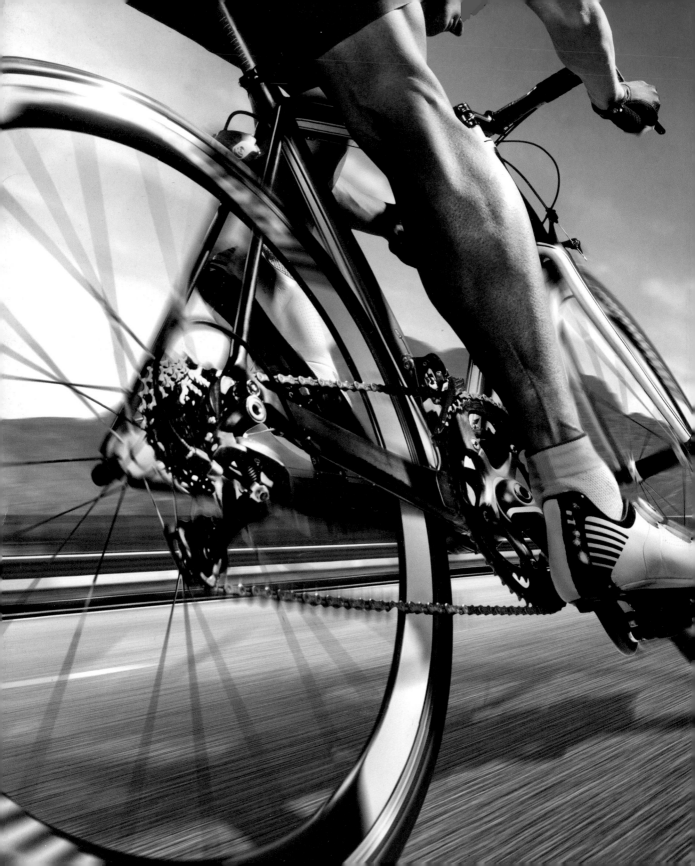

Phil Burt and Martin Evans

STRENGTH AND CONDITIONING FOR CYCLISTS

Off The Bike Conditioning for Performance and Life

BLOOMSBURY SPORT

LONDON · OXFORD · NEW YORK · NEW DELHI · SYDNEY

BLOOMSBURY SPORT

Bloomsbury Publishing Plc
50 Bedford Square, London,
WC1B 3DP, UK

BLOOMSBURY, BLOOMSBURY SPORT
and the Diana logo are trademarks of
Bloomsbury Publishing Plc

First published in Great Britain 2018

A catalogue record for this book is
available from the British Library

Library of Congress Cataloging-in-
Publication data has been applied for

ISBN: PB: 978-1-4729-4013-1
    eBook: 978-1-4729-4012-4

2 4 6 8 10 9 7 5 3 1

Typeset in PMN Caecilia and Lato
Designed by Austin Taylor
Printed and bound in China by
    Toppan Leefung Printing

To find out more about our authors
and books visit www.bloomsbury.com
and sign up for our newsletters

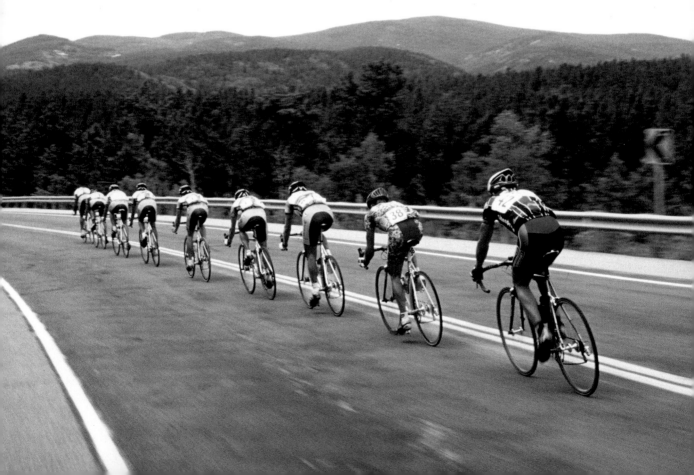

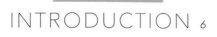

CONTENTS

INTRODUCTION

Many cycling training manuals fall far short of the mark when prescribing off the bike training routines. There are certainly proven performance gains to be had from off the bike conditioning for all cyclists but not in the simplistic way that's often presented.

The problem is that, with one-size-fits-all generic routines, crucial steps in laying the foundations of conditioning are ignored. If you imagine building your fitness as being analogous to building a house, without good foundations any further floors, no matter how well built, are always destined eventually to fail. This failure could be a lack of progress or potentially developing imbalances and injuries. Yes, if you go to the gym and start performing dead lifts and barbell squats, as commonly prescribed in many generic cycling-specific gym routines, you'll probably make some apparent strength gains but, without the foundations that'll allow you to perform these movements safely and effectively, those gains are fundamentally compromised and flawed.

BUILDING A STABLE PYRAMID

Cycling fitness, and all conditioning, can be thought of as a pyramid. A pyramid is only stable if it has a broad base with your actual fitness on the bike as just the capstone on the top. At the bottom (Level 1) are general physical qualities. This broad base encompasses range of movement (ROM) and control through that range. For example, when you are lying on your back on the floor, how far can you raise your leg while keeping it straight? If you're unable to elevate it to 75 degrees, you're lacking range of movement through your hamstrings and hips. Now try lowering it. Can you do this under control, without the small of your back leaving

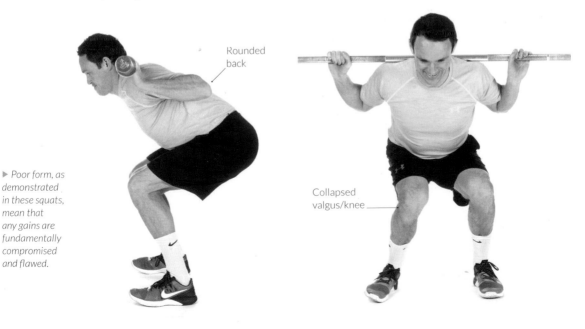

Rounded back

Collapsed valgus/knee

▶ *Poor form, as demonstrated in these squats, mean that any gains are fundamentally compromised and flawed.*

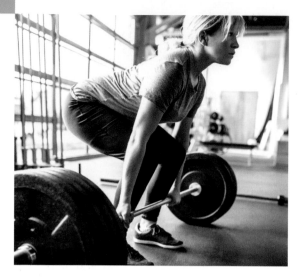

▲ *Maximal power, which can transfer to your cycling performance, can be enhanced with gym work.*

the floor? If no, you lack control through the range you have. This in itself may not seem like a big deal but such limitations have major implications on your ability to perform lifts and even to perform movements associated with everyday life. Next (Level 2) are the physical qualities related to cycling but that are not necessarily developed on the bike. These could include maximal power, which you may have enhanced with work in the gym, or a range of motion that allows you to hold an aggressive time trial position. Finally, we come to the top of the pyramid (Level 3) and the cycling-specific fitness that you develop on the bike. Unfortunately, for a huge number of cyclists, including, until fairly recently, top-level elite riders, the capstone was all they really focused on, with little regard for the crucial layers below. Miss or neglect the steps that will develop these foundations, or just ride your bike, and no matter how fast you can cycle, your pyramid is unstable and destined to topple.

Another way to think of this is in terms of moderators versus mediators. Moderating factors, such as good strength, optimal range of movement and high levels of adaptability, form that strong stable base of your pyramid. Mediating factors are issues that can lead to injury, breakdown or poor adaptation. Prior injury history or a narrow training focus can be thought of as mediating factors.

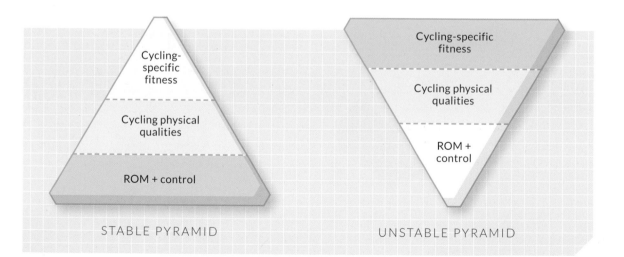

Cycling-specific fitness

Cycling physical qualities

ROM + control

STABLE PYRAMID

Cycling-specific fitness

Cycling physical qualities

ROM + control

UNSTABLE PYRAMID

The interaction between moderators and mediators determines how an athlete will respond to a given training stimulus or block of training. Traditionally, the approach to trying to predict this outcome has been extremely reductionist but, in both studies and when working with athletes, this just doesn't work. An example of this is hamstring tightness, which was viewed as a predictor for injury. Unfortunately, it just doesn't correlate and it's possible to have extremely tight but also very strong hamstrings. The reason this reductionist approach doesn't work is that human beings are extremely complex systems. Even with incredible amounts of data and the most powerful supercomputers, we're unable to reliably predict the weather more than a couple of days ahead, so how can we even consider trying to apply one-size-fits-all predictions to the equally complex human body? There are just too many moderators and mediators interacting and impacting on the final result of any intervention.

Everyone is different and we like to talk about riders in terms of micro-adjusters and macro-absorbers. Micro-adjusters are those riders who are extremely sensitive to change, can easily slip into a state of maladaptation and are more prone to injury. An example of this type of rider is Ben Swift – he'll notice the smallest change in his bike set-up and has had to work extremely hard on his off the bike conditioning to improve his resilience. At the extreme macro-absorber end of the spectrum is Geraint Thomas. You can throw the kitchen sink at him in training and he's just able to soak it up. Put him on someone else's bike during a Grand Tour stage and even if the set-up is significantly different to his, he can ride

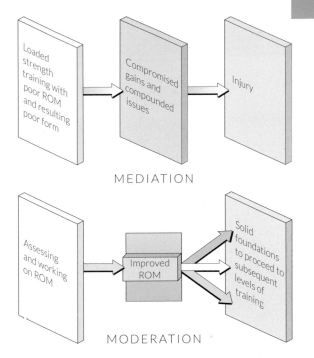

MEDIATION

MODERATION

▲ Examples of mediation and moderation and their potential future impacts on training. Adapted from Gabbett et al 2017.

it and hardly notice. At school, there was probably a child – you may have been lucky and it was you – who was just naturally good at everything. They would be a macro-absorber.

Whether it's how you respond to training, a predisposition to injury or your medical history, what works for one rider might not be appropriate for you. A great example of this was Ed Clancy recovering from back injury. We put him in an altitude chamber to allow him to ride with a really low load but, at the same time, stress his heart and lungs. All the studies and past experience said that this should have worked but the simple fact was that it didn't. He got worse and worse, and although it felt counter-intuitive, we had to find a different approach for him. Similarly, the infamously brutal pre-Tour Mount Teide altitude training camp took both Sir Bradley Wiggins and Chris Froome to Tour de France-winning performance levels. However, the same camp has seen other riders simply crumble under the load. No one size fits all, and although we can make intelligent and educated guesses about outcomes, we have to be flexible and holistic in our approach.

If we can't predict exactly how moderators and mediators are going to interact, what can we do? The solution, as much as possible, is to stack your deck in favour of moderators. This means training hard but also training smart and building a wide base of conditioning. You might not be lucky enough to be a natural macro-absorber but, by working hard on developing that stable pyramid and not neglecting off the bike training, you can significantly improve the odds in your favour.

WHO'S IT FOR?

A wide range of factors, including genetics, injury history, activity levels and even our work, mean that very few individuals have the range of movement, control and strength to go straight into loaded strength training movements. This isn't a criticism or a condemnation of your ability. You can be assured that Olympic champions and Tour de France winners have exactly the same issues. Knowing how to assess and address these issues, with the input, knowledge and expertise of medical and conditioning experts, has largely only been accessible to elite or wealthy athletes. Using this book, however, we will provide that expertise and guide you through an effective and easy-to-follow process that will ensure you can build those solid foundations,

know when it's appropriate to move on to more demanding exercises and undoubtedly make you a stronger, more robust and resilient cyclist.

An assessment based on the screening process used with the Great Britain Cycling Team is at the heart of the process. The tests it uses will quickly identify your strengths and weaknesses and then guide you to exactly the exercises you need to do. It results in a highly personalised routine that's completely appropriate to your abilities and limitations at that moment in time. By working on the exercises that your assessment prescribed and then retesting, you can be confident that you're progressing and challenging your body in a safe and effective way.

It's appropriate for a wide range of cyclists, from complete novices and injured riders returning to activity to ambitious, experienced riders looking for that competitive edge. You won't require expensive equipment and the majority of riders can make significant progress and noticeable improvements in their own homes without the need for a gym membership. It's not a get-fit-quick fix for cycling strength but, if followed correctly and maintained, it will give you a valuable broad base of conditioning that will benefit you both on and off the bike for years to come. It's a tool that you can continually come back to and use throughout your cycling career and even beyond. If during your main event build-up or race season you dial back your off the bike conditioning, simply reassess once you want to reintroduce it, find where you are on the plan and re-enter at that level. You might find you have regressed while

▶ *A well designed and individually tailored off the bike conditioning plan is appropriate for riders of all levels.*

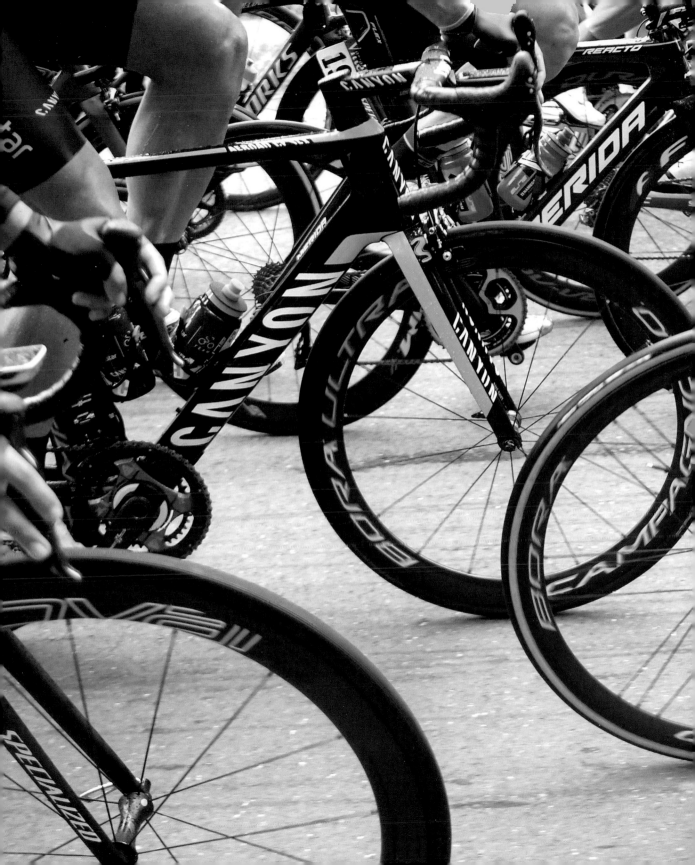

focusing more on your bike, but you will know, by following the progression of this book, that you can successfully rebuild and rebalance your pyramid.

You might think that such an individualised and focused approach is only for full-time professional athletes but that couldn't be further from the truth. It's arguable that regular off the bike conditioning work is even more important and beneficial to part-time riders than for full-time professionals. Referring back to the pyramid of conditioning that we talked about earlier in the chapter, cycling on its own, in terms of movement and conditioning, is a very narrow activity and won't give you that crucial all-round athletic broad base. Without this base, your layers above, including your cycling, will be limited and compromised. If you focus solely on cycling, your pyramid will be inverted, which, as we've previously discussed, isn't stable or sustainable.

Let's be clear, there is solid research evidence that off the bike conditioning work will undoubtedly make you faster on the bike (Mujika et al., 2016). You'll increase the physical capabilities of your muscles and, in doing so, the amount of force you're able

to apply to your pedals. The most obvious benefit of this will be in those village sign sprints or battles for the top of a climb, but it'll also improve your cycling across intensities. By improving the maximal capabilities of your muscles, specifically the rate at which force is applied, you'll be more economical when riding sub-maximally. This will improve your efficiency and so your ability to ride harder for longer. A good analogy is driving on the motorway at 70 mph. A car with a top speed of 160 mph will be far more efficient at 70 mph than a car that maxes out at 90 mph. These benefits have been strongly related to performance in a 40-minute time

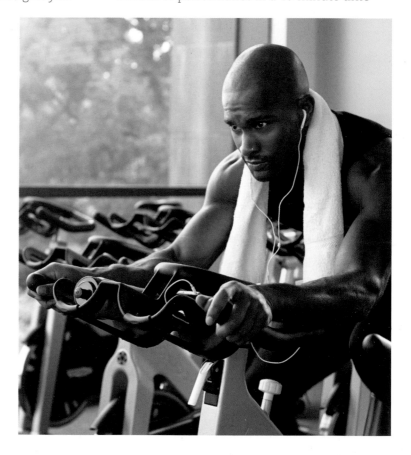

▶ If you're spending time in the gym, some focused off the bike work is probably better for your cycling and sanity than grinding away on a stationary bike.

trial (Ronnestad et al., 2015). It has also been shown to increase 30-second power output in elite cyclists (Ronnestad et al., 2010) and 5-minute all out performance following 185 minutes' cycling (Ronnestad et al., 2011).

However, it'll also deliver a host of other benefits, the most important being your robustness and resilience to injury. Unlike a professional cyclist, who will mostly be either riding their bike or sitting on the sofa, you have to lift your kids out of the car, carry shopping, do DIY and work in the garden. By improving your general physical qualities or general movement capabilities and capacities, you'll be more able to cope with the twists and bends that life throws at you. Less time spent injured means more time out on your bike.

You can think about how your body moves in terms of degrees of freedom. Many cyclists have very limited degrees of freedom. If your degrees of freedom are limited, such as extremely tight hips and lower back, this can definitely impact directly on your cycling. You'll only be able to pedal and generate power in one limited sphere of movement and, in doing this thousands of times in one ride and often to exhaustion, overuse injuries and imbalances tend to develop. By becoming strong through a wider range of movements and developing more degrees of freedom, your body isn't limited to one power production pathway, increasing your resilience both on and off the bike.

Finally, off the bike conditioning work can make you healthier. It can slow and even reverse the loss of muscle mass associated with ageing, improving health and strength and facilitating weight control. It'll also improve bone health, specifically bone density, which is an issue even for Grand Tour riders.

BREAKING WITH TRADITION

Professional cycling is a sport that's steeped in tradition. Up until surprisingly recently, riders trained and ate in a way that would have felt very familiar to cyclists from as far back as the 1950s. Whether it was riding thousands of kilometres, never pushing beyond conversational pace and twiddling a tiny gear in the name of winter base training or getting up at four in the morning to tuck into a steak before a race, that's how it'd always been done. These methods were never questioned and, as riders retired and became directeurs sportifs or coaches, these sacraments were handed on to the next generation. Off the bike conditioning work was viewed at best as a bit of fun for the off season and often involved little more than a bit of cross-country skiing or a token number of ill-conceived and poorly attended gym sessions at training camps. The argument was that cyclists ride bikes, so the best and pretty much only training they should do is ride their bikes. However, as the academic discipline of sports science became more established and more voices started to challenge cycling's dogmas, things slowly started to change. More progressive teams, such as the Great Britain Cycling Team and Team Sky, threw out the rule book, looked outside of cycling's closed shop and revolutionised the sport. No stone was left unturned in the quest for improved performance. At the end of a five- or six-hour Grand Tour stage, finishing on a mountain summit or in a flat-out bunch sprint, the accepted protocol would be a can of Coke and then straight off to the hotel or, if you were required, podium or press duties. Despite the

Pain

Lower back pain can be a normal part of adaptation to a new activity, whether on the bike or as a result of completing a heavy lifting session in resistance training. A sore lower back isn't necessarily a bad thing, worrying as it might seem at the time.

Pain can be incredibly useful. If you go to lift a casserole out of the oven but forget your oven glove, pain tells you to let go quickly before you burn your hand too badly. This is a useful pain – it alerts you to prevent further damage. Similarly, if you watch a dog rehabilitate themselves from an injured paw, pain lets them know how much they can load their bad leg and, by gradually increasing the weight they put through it, they progressively rebuild strength and function bit by bit. It's only when pain becomes chronic that it becomes non-useful and a problem.

Returning to lower back pain, as it's so prevalent in the Western world, the common approach to an injured back is to rest up and to avoid the movement that led to the injury. This is correct at the very beginning but only for a short period of time, days not weeks. The problem is the advice encourages people to continue with the avoidance of moving. The pain might ease but at the same time the back de-conditions and becomes even more vulnerable. Often the pain then continues or worsens, even though the original issue has healed up and there's no remaining pathology. In the case of chronic pain, the body is generating pain messages for no good reason at all. Even though resting up might seem like the best approach, more often than not, after the initial period of inflammation, moving and loading the structures in a controlled way is the best route to a full recovery.

Chronic pain, including the lower back, can be a vicious circle. It's easy to fall into a mindset where you're scared of doing the things that would do the most good – moving and exercise – because you think they're going to hurt and potentially cause more damage. Not doing anything makes the pain worse and you get locked into something called a pain behaviour pattern. A great example of the opposite mindset is Sir Chris Hoy, and it's one of the possible reasons behind his six Olympic gold medals. He'd come in sore from previous training but rather than saying he couldn't lift in the gym, he'd ask what he could do to allow him to lift.

We're not suggesting that you adopt a 'no pain, no gain' approach and if you are suffering from worrying acute or long-standing chronic pain, obtaining professional medical advice is definitely wise. However, rather than focusing on what you *can't* do because of the pain, try to get into the mindset of asking what you *can* do with it.

Another type of pain that you're likely to come across, especially if you're new to off the bike training or it's your first weights session of the off season, is delayed onset muscle soreness or DOMS. If you do a workout or an exercise that's new to your muscles, you'll stress them, causing them to adapt and repair. Part of this adaptation and repair is a degree of inflammation, and this can lead to pain or soreness occurring 12–24 hours after the session and lasting for 24–48 hours. It's not a bad thing and, although it may cause you to struggle with stairs, you shouldn't be to trying reduce it as it's part of the adaptation process that will lead to you getting stronger. Therefore, there's no need for ice baths because the goal is to stress your body to stimulate a response – to get stronger. The DOMS is the stimulus working and your body adapting and, by doing anything to reduce this response, you're effectively contradicting the aim of the training you're doing. Ice baths are useful in contact sports such as rugby, where contusion injuries cause DOMS like stiffness and soreness. If you have a bad case of DOMS, probably the best thing you can do is to go for a very light spin on your bike.

It can sometimes be difficult to determine whether pain is a genuine injury or an appropriate and natural response to the training you've done. A good rule of thumb is simply to check whether you've got the pain on both sides or just one side of your body. If both of your hamstrings are sore and you did some hard sprints on the bike or lifted the day before, it's probably just DOMS. If only one is sore and the pain is more localised, it's more likely you may have a restriction or something that may need working through, perhaps with professional medical guidance.

▼ *Cycling can be painful but that pain has to be appropriate.*

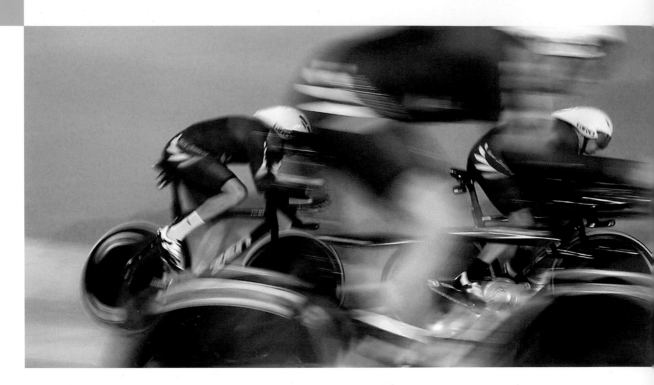

intensity of the final effort of the stage, little or no thought was given to any aspect of post-ride recovery. Team Sky were looked on as eccentrics when they had their riders performing gradual warm-downs on turbos after such stages, but now it's accepted practice by all teams and it's hard to imagine it not happening. The team also transported their own bedding from hotel to hotel. Monotonous mountains of pasta were replaced with protein-rich meals, vegetable juices and fish oils. Such practices were viewed with as much suspicion as the post-ride warm-down and initially ridiculed too but, as Tour wins and Olympic medals started to mount up, the cycling world started to take note. The same process has happened with off the bike conditioning and, despite the academic research into its benefits to cycling having been

available for a number of years, it's only now being seen as an essential tool for all riders.

LESSONS FROM THE TRACK

One of the key components of the model for success of the Great Britain Cycling Team was focusing on the timed events on the track. These events, without the unpredictable and tactical elements of bunch or road racing, could be accurately assessed and planned for. They could be distilled down to the numbers required to win and then worked towards by combining all performance gains offered by training, nutrition and equipment. One of our most successful disciplines on the track has been the Team Pursuit, but over the last three Olympic cycles this event has changed

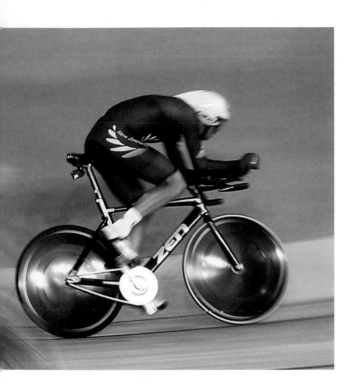

◀ *Working in the gym for the team pursuit, riders started to see benefits to their performance on the road too.*

massively. It has become faster and faster, blurring the line between sprint and endurance events. Despite the event lasting around 4 minutes, definitely qualifying it physiologically as endurance, the riders have to produce 15–30-second near maximal efforts when on the front and generate huge amounts of power to get the big gears turning from the start. Gym work has always been a massive part of the training regime of track sprinters, often jokingly referred to as weightlifters who occasionally ride bikes, and, with sprint and endurance squads and coaches working so closely together on the track, cross-pollination of ideas started to occur. Progressive endurance coaches on the Great Britain Cycling Team, such as Paul Manning, Dan Hunt and Matt Parker, started asking us if there were potentially gains to be made in the gym for the

road riders coming in to ride the Team Pursuit. Initially the approach was 'softly softly' and probably slightly watered down, due to the spectre of tradition still casting a shadow of fear concerning injuries, but, especially after the London Olympics, gym work has been a cornerstone in the training plan of the endurance squad. With most of the riders also competing on the road, they inevitably started to see benefits to that aspect of their riding too and the idea of the use of off the bike conditioning slowly started to pervade the professional peloton. A great example of the cross-pollination of ideas from the track to the road was Sir Bradley Wiggins's assault on the World Time Trial Championships in 2014. In the lead-up to this event, he went through a 12-week block with the specific goal of making him bigger and stronger, in comparison with his stage-racing physique, for the 47.10km Ponferrada course. It worked, with him winning by a massive 26-second margin over time-trialling legend Tony Martin.

IS IT WORTH SACRIFICING RIDING TIME FOR?

With work, family and other demands on their time, many amateur cyclists are understandably concerned about dedicating any of their precious riding time, let alone two or three hours a week, to off the bike training. Hopefully, as you've bought this book, you're already interested in optimising your off the

What about the 'core'?

It might surprise you to be reading a book about off the bike conditioning and, so far, to have heard no mention of the word 'core' or the vital importance of developing core stability. Unfortunately, the terms 'core' and 'core stability' are incredibly misunderstood and their misuse is responsible for an awful lot of riders, and other athletes and people exercising purely for health-related goals, wasting an awful lot of their precious time. It's a real shame that these terms have been so abused as it's really important for humans, having four independent limbs, to be able to control the central anchor for all of them, namely the trunk. Yet somehow, rather than seeing the trunk and its deeply complex interaction with our limbs and the rest of the body as a big picture, the fitness industry and health media seem to be obsessed with isolated muscles.

This erroneous reductionist approach is often taken to the extreme. In many instances, when people talk about the core they are referring to specific muscles that are thought to be especially important for spinal stabilisation, in particular the transverse abdominis (TrA).

In the 1990s, research in Australia suggested that weakness in the TrA was responsible for the majority of lower back pain. With back pain such a prevalent complaint in modern society, the physiotherapy world adopted this universal 'cure all', followed in turn by the fitness industry, and the core stability trend began. Small, precise and isolated movements that targeted the TrA were not only being prescribed for people suffering from back injuries, but also for fitness enthusiasts and athletes searching for performance gains and injury prevention. It is now more commonly accepted that many different muscles of the trunk contribute to its function and that the mechanisms for stabilisation of the trunk may change according to the task being performed. For example, the trunk is going to be working very differently during a dead lift compared with when you're riding your bike. Therefore, how we view and approach training the trunk asks the same question as any performance problem: what are you trying to achieve?

Are you trying to rehabilitate your trunk after surgery or injury? If so, then some commonly prescribed core-training strategies that try to isolate certain muscle groups and train them to continuously contract – for example, hollowing the abdominals – may not be appropriate. These 'bracing'-type movements, so popular with core enthusiasts, may not be the answer as these muscles often work in a reflexive manner, rather than being continuously contracted in readiness.

▼ *'Core Stability' isn't the panacea of well-being that the health and fitness industry sometimes portray it to be.*

Going back to the lower back pain study referred to earlier, the onset of TrA activity was delayed by just 20 milliseconds, which is beyond conscious control. Therefore, training these muscles to brace and continuously contract isn't addressing the root cause of the problem, namely the timing of the reactive contraction, and therefore is likely to be ineffective and could be potentially harmful.

Lower back soreness, discomfort or tightness during and after cycling is often thought of as being indicative of weak 'core' muscles and, because of this, many riders spend huge amounts of time performing exercises, often lying down with very small amounts of movement, in an attempt to correct this. However, it's often the case that lower back soreness on the bike is more likely to be caused by a poor bike fit, a simple lack of conditioning or a bewildering combination of many factors.

If you ran a marathon for the first time, you'd expect to feel some discomfort during it and certainly afterwards. Similarly, if you're used to riding for an hour or two at a certain intensity, and then you ramp it up to three hours or push the pace, you're going to feel it. Because of the flexed forward position of cycling, the musculature of your trunk and lower back is having to work hard, and that's probably why you end up feeling a bit stiff and sore. Some mobility work would help, some strength work would help, and more time and structured training on the bike would definitely help. What's probably not going to help are hours of 'core strengthening' exercises. Immediately there will be riders rising up at this statement, convinced that a bout of core strengthening cured their cycling lower back pain, but the reality is that the 'cure' probably came from rest from the aggravating activities that could have been leading to the soreness, and just the simple healing effect of time.

Lower back pain, or any pain, can be symptomatic of adaptation. If we return to our rider heading out for a three-hour ride, if he carried on riding for three hours, his body would adapt, including his lower back musculature, and he would be able to ride for that duration with less discomfort. The caveat for this, though, is that everything else in the system of bike and rider is good and functioning properly. This includes his bike fit and the overall conditioning of his body. If, say, he completed our assessment described in Chapter 1 and consistently failed the active straight leg raise, due to tight or restricted hip flexors, this is a flaw in the system. In this case the adaptation would be compromised, and this is why an all-over and personalised approach to conditioning, not just cycling and certainly not poorly prescribed core exercises, is essential.

An overly reductionist approach to core muscles and lower back pain fails because it tries to isolate one factor for being responsible for a complex and multifactorial issue. As already discussed earlier in the chapter, when talking about mediators and moderators, this approach simply doesn't work for a complex system such as the human body.

Whether we like it or not, the term 'core' is here to stay and means so many different things to many different people. It's the authors' opinion that we're unlikely to change this, but we should strive to discover better and clearer ways of describing the trunk's obviously vital role in how human beings move and perform.

It would be great if we could recognise that trunk stability, strength and mobility are of equal importance in generating movement of our limbs and the trunk itself, and protecting us from pain and injury. We have to stop trying to oversimplify and reduce complex systems and complex issues, and applying one-stop blanket and narrow solutions.

bike conditioning but it's still worthwhile to allay those concerns. Firstly, as we've just explained, off the bike conditioning will improve your cycling performance and, in the long term, will save you time off the bike in the future due to injury. Secondly, it's about planning and prioritising your training. We're definitely not saying that you have to go to the gym religiously for three hours, week in and week out, for the rest of your cycling life. There will be phases, such as in the final build-up to a big sportive or during your racing season, when off the bike work will be minimal and only serve as a maintenance function. However, before those big endurance builds or competition blocks, off the bike work can help to prepare the body and build resilience for the hard on the bike work to come. For many riders, this will mean that the winter is a good time to focus on gym work; it also gets you out of the bad weather. However, if your priority is cyclo-cross or the track season, your 'off

season' may be the spring or autumn. It's a case of identifying your main goals, prioritising them and looking to see where you would benefit most from a dedicated block of gym work. We've no doubt that all riders would benefit from off the bike conditioning work; it's just a case of working out when it'd be optimal for you and your cycling goals. This is no different to how we work with the riders on the Great Britain Cycling Team and they accept that, at certain times of year, their performance on the bike may suffer because of the work they're doing in the gym or even because they're deeply fatigued from a big road block. However, they know that, as their training moves on towards key events, this work is the foundation for their successes. This is the mindset you have to learn to adopt. Don't be surprised if your performance on the Sunday club run does suffer during an off the bike conditioning block, but know that it'll pay dividends when you hit that first sportive in

High reps for riding

One of the things you commonly hear when people (even supposedly qualified coaches) are talking about weight training for cycling is that you should be doing low weight and high reps as this mimics the high rep demand of pedalling.

This is incorrect on two levels. The first is that you're not trying to mimic cycling in the gym, you're trying to change the nature of the muscle and then apply that stronger muscle to cycling. For example, even if you do 5 sets of 50 reps with a super light load, that's still only 250 reps. This

may seem a lot but when you consider that you'll achieve that number of pedal strokes in under 3 minutes of riding, the argument of high reps to mimic the demands of cycling just doesn't stack up. Secondly, in order to improve the force that you can apply through your pedals, you have to be applying a sufficient load to the muscles. Sets of 20 reps or more simply don't apply enough of a load to stimulate the changes in the muscle that result in greater force output. Low-weight and high-rep work is, at best, an ineffective waste of time and, as it often involves poor form and rushed movement, can compound existing limitations.

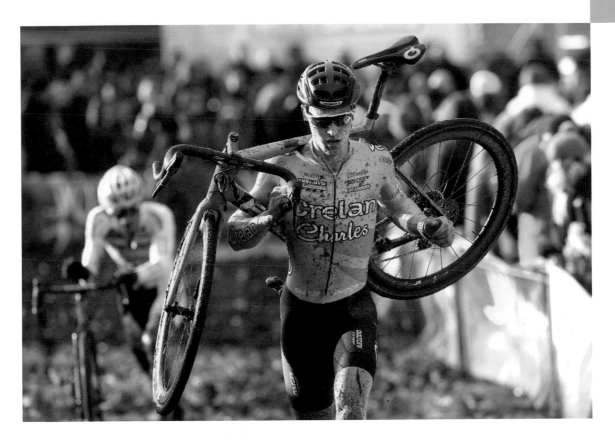

the spring. A good training plan should be constantly progressing and worked back from your main goals. If you're repeatedly doing the same thing, week in, week out, and always expecting to continuously improve, you will quickly reach a plateau of performance and stay there. Millions of years of evolution have made our bodies incredibly efficient and, unless we give them good reason to change, they won't commit valuable resources to doing so. These reasons are the training stimuli that you provide and if they don't constantly shock and challenge your body, you'll stay stuck in a

▲ *Although the winter is often seen as the time for off the bike work, if you're racing cyclo-cross, spring or autumn may be more appropriate.*

training rut. Focusing more on your off the bike conditioning may mean you operate below that plateau in terms of cycling for a period of time. However, when you effectively release the handbrake of the strength training you've done and refocus on the bike, expect to smash through that plateau and hit new levels of performance.

Also, as you'll soon realise when you go through the initial assessment, there are a number of stages to go through before you reach the sort of loaded exercises that can potentially acutely blunt your cycling form. Many of the exercises that we prescribe can be a permanent feature in your training routine and can be used pre-lifting, when and if you progress to loaded exercises in the gym, and pre/post-training in general, including riding. For example, the posterior thigh opener stretch (see Chapter 2) would be brilliant for many riders after a hard session in the saddle or if you've been sitting at your desk or driving all day, before you head out on your bike.

We'll go into more details on how to schedule your off the bike conditioning later in the book and, if you are especially pressed for time, we will always guide you towards the exercises that will have the greatest impact for you.

With regard to frequency and volume of off the bike conditioning, this will vary depending on your phase of training, level or function and your goals. During the earlier stages of the plan, where you are primarily working on mobility, daily bite-sized sessions working on your areas of weakness could prove most effective. However, scheduling in a few dedicated and focused 20–30-minute sessions would also be a good idea to ensure progress. This sort of work won't have any negative effects on your riding – if anything, it will be positive – and won't require you to factor in any dedicated recovery time.

If you do move on to loaded exercises, most of the research would suggest that for the physiological adaptations to take place, a training block should be at least 8–12 weeks. You would ideally be looking to perform 2–3 dedicated off the bike conditioning sessions per week during this time period. You should allow 48 hours' recovery between sessions. You can obviously carry on cycling during these blocks but it's important that your riding does not impact on the quality of your off the bike training. Don't try to pack everything in

together; organise your training and focus on the main goal of the specific training block.

HOW DO I KNOW WHICH EXERCISES TO DO?

The key factor, which many books on cycling training neglect, is that every cyclist is different. They will prescribe a generic off the bike routine with little or no thought to your individual strengths and weaknesses. A classic example is that almost every cycling strength routine you see will prescribe a barbell back squat. Yes, this is a great exercise, but the vast majority of cyclists lack the trunk strength, all-round flexibility and technique to perform it safely and effectively. When riders enter the Great Britain Cycling Team Academy, we can see almost straight away that certain exercises won't be suitable for certain of them or that there are movement or postural issues that'll need working on before they progress to lifting weights. All riders are different, even at the top level. We've already talked about the differences between micro-adjuster Ben Swift and macro-absorber Geraint Thomas. The off the bike programmes they'd need to do would be very different. Ben had to dedicate a lot of time to off the bike conditioning and rectifying movement and postural issues. By doing this, he has made himself into a far more robust and successful rider than if he'd just carried on riding his bike.

In this book, the starting point is a self-assessment, which determines your areas of strength and weakness.

The self-assessment is inspired by the same screening that all riders entering the Great

Britain Cycling Team undertake. Along with the physical tests, it also investigates lifestyle, past training and injuries, and even family histories. This self-assessment will allow you to determine your individual requirements, limitations and risks, providing a personal prescription of exercises most suited to you. Once you have completed the self-assessment, the book will tell you which particular exercises are key to you, the sets and reps you'll need to perform, and then how to plan in your sessions and organise your training.

With constant reassessment, you'll be focusing on specific and personalised goals, building that base of your pyramid and progressing through the plan. Your routine will never remain static as it evolves along with the progress you make. Depending on your starting level, you'll move from mobilisation and control to range, and finally on to movement capacity and actual lifting. Every step will contribute towards you becoming more resilient and a stronger, faster and more successful cyclist.

WHAT EQUIPMENT WILL I NEED?

Based on the results of your assessment, you will enter the programme at different levels. At the first level, which is essentially developing control through range of movement, the equipment requirement will be minimal. At most you will need a mat, foam roller, trigger point ball, resistance bands, dumbbells or a kettlebell and maybe a bench or step. For a large number of cyclists, achieving the physical capabilities of this level will represent a significant improvement.

Further levels will require a greater amount of equipment as the movements are loaded. This may require you to join a gym to allow you to access the necessary equipment and loads.

It's important to realise, though, that the majority of cyclists stand to benefit greatly from the control through motion and bodyweight work of the earlier levels. Just by performing and progressing these movements, they can significantly reduce their injury risk potential.

Will it make me bulky and slower uphill?

The primary goals of the programme are to improve your general physical qualities and general movement capabilities, and then to develop peak and the rate of muscular force production. Gaining some lean muscle mass might be a by-product of this but muscles can certainly become stronger without becoming heavier. In fact, one study of elite cyclists found that they gained thigh muscle mass without an increase in body mass (Ronnestad et al., 2010). It's also incredibly difficult to gain significant muscle bulk even if you want to. The lengths that bodybuilders go to illustrate this, and one of the first steps they take is to minimise all aerobic and endurance work from their training. If you're combining your off the bike conditioning work with your cycling, you're definitely not going to turn into the Hulk. Additionally, unless you already have excellent functional movement, you're not going to be hitting heavy weights for a while.

CHAPTER SUMMARY

All riders are individuals
Every cyclist is an individual and, in the same way that power and heart-rate training zones, training sessions and overall training plans should be tailored to the individual, the same applies to off the bike conditioning. It is only by first discovering an individual's strengths, limitations and weaknesses that an appropriate and effective off the bike conditioning routine can be prescribed.

Building a broad base of conditioning
Your overall conditioning can be thought of as a pyramid with often neglected physical qualities, such as range of movement (ROM) and control through that range, forming its base. Your actual cycling fitness and performance should just be the capstone on the top. For the vast majority of cyclists, their pyramid is inverted or has a very narrow base. This means that all of the layers of fitness above are unstable and, often due to injury, liable to fail. By investing time in building a broad and solid base, all of the layers above will be more stable. This will make you less prone to injury and will directly enhance your cycling performance.

Pain
Like constructing a training plan, pain is massively individual. It can be incredibly useful, stopping us from burning a hand, or debilitating, as with chronic lower back pain. Seeking professional advice is always wise but, in the majority of cases, after the initial inflammation of an injury, managed and progressive activity, rather than rest, is the optimum path to recovery.

Ditching the dogma
Cycling is a sport with training dogma deeply rooted in the past. It's only in recent years that this 'how it's always been done' mindset has been challenged. Off the bike conditioning has been one of the most significant areas of progress and where once it received scant attention, it's now seen as essential for all top cyclists. Even if you're not embarking on a Grand Tour campaign or on the hunt for an Olympic gold, you can improve not only your cycling but your overall health and resilience to injury.

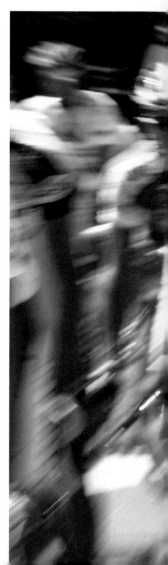

Time well spent

We know how precious those hours you spend on your bike are to you, so we wouldn't be advising you to sacrifice some of them unless we were sure of the benefits. Especially during the earlier stages of the process, when you're focusing on that broad base of mobility, daily bite-sized chunks can be really effective. As you progress on to loaded exercises, you will learn how to programme blocks of this type of training into your cycling year to maximise the positive effects on your cycling.

Minimal kit

The equipment required to work through the majority of the plan is minimal and you certainly won't require a gym membership. It is only if and when you progress on to more advanced loaded movements, which isn't necessarily needed for the vast majority of endurance-focused riders, that you'll require the equipment typically found in a gym.

▼ *All riders, no matter what level, stand to benefit from structured and individually focused off the bike training.*

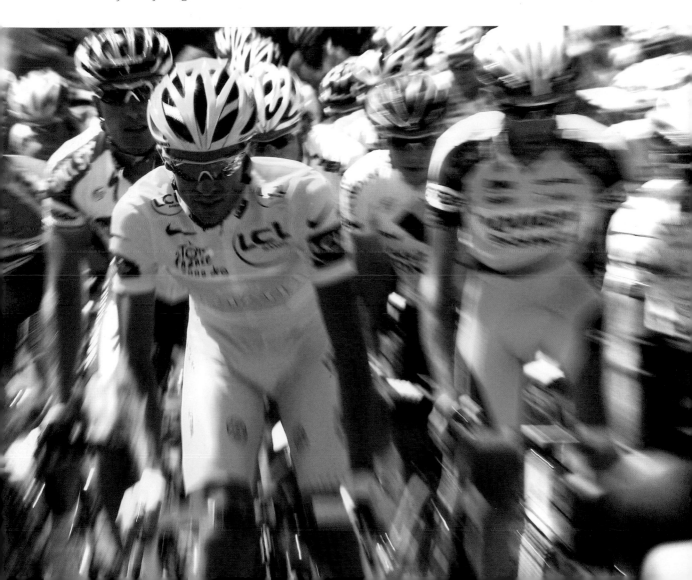

THE
ASSESSMENT

As we've previously established, many cycling training manuals provide a one-size-fits-all generic off the bike conditioning routine. At best, such routines are ineffective or a waste of the rider's valuable time but, in some cases, they can be dangerous and actually lead to injury.

As we said in the introduction, cycling, in terms of movement and conditioning, is a very narrow activity and, as a result, many riders are limited in terms of their movement capabilities and physical qualities. Setting them off blindly on a routine of back squats or dead lifts, for example, is potentially disastrous. It's only by ascertaining the current level and limitations of a rider that an appropriate series of exercises can be prescribed. This is why an assessment is such an essential part of off the bike conditioning.

This assessment, which is fundamental to the book, is based on what we put all riders through when they join the Great Britain Cycling Team programme. If the assessment uncovers any areas of weakness, remedying that area will be their number one priority. This could mean less time lifting in the gym, or even less time on the bike for a period of time, but we know that in terms of the longevity and success of their career, it's an essential investment to make.

Equally, you too can be sure that by determining your individual strengths and weaknesses, the off the bike training you do is relevant and effective for your needs. If we're honest with ourselves, we all tend to prefer to work to our strengths. There are probably cycling workouts that you gravitate towards because you're good at them and therefore enjoy them more. If you're a climber, you probably enjoy hilly rides, whereas if you're a bigger rouleur, you'll tend towards flatter riding. However, in the majority of cases, it's by identifying and focusing on our weaknesses that we stand to make the greatest gains. This definitely applies to off the bike conditioning and the weaknesses that the assessment identifies should be thought of as potential low-hanging fruit for performance and resilience gains. You'll be able to maintain your current strengths while working on them but, by doing so, you'll build that wide base of your conditioning pyramid and become a stronger and more rounded and successful cyclist.

▼ The assessment is like an MOT for your body, finding the specific areas that you need to work on.

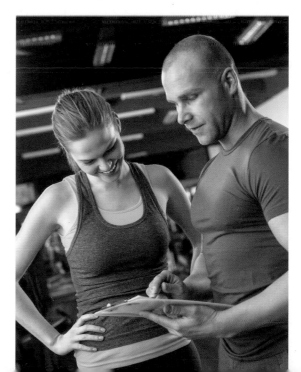

ARE THE ASSESSMENT AND ROUTINES RIGHT FOR ME?

It's important to realise that this isn't an assessment of your ability to ride a bike – we're assuming you're able to do that already – but an assessment of whether you can safely and effectively conduct resistance and strength training. By gauging and assessing your current level it's possible to determine your pathway for developing your movement capabilities where most needed.

It's not a one-time pass or fail assessment, either; you'll constantly revisit the assessment, moving through the levels and evolving and improving as an athlete. You can view it as being analogous to maintaining your bike. You'll check over your bike before each ride and, if necessary, put some air in the tyres, tighten the headset or lube the chain. If the bike is broken, there are simple things you can do to make it work better. View the assessment in the same way as a pre-ride bike check and the exercises as body maintenance tasks.

The diagram below shows a normal distribution curve of cyclists. At either end are the relatively small groups to whom this book doesn't apply. The first group are those riders who, for medical reasons, have specialist needs that are beyond the remit of this book. At the other end of the curve are world-class athletes who will already include high-level strength and conditioning work in their training programmes. In the middle are the vast majority of cyclists, from novice sportive riders to competitive racers, who stand to benefit from this book.

You should be pain-free before undertaking the assessment or, if you do currently have an injury or suffer from pain or discomfort, either on or off the bike, you should consult with an appropriate health professional. They

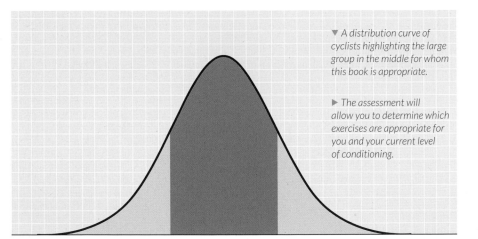

▼ A distribution curve of cyclists highlighting the large group in the middle for whom this book is appropriate.

▶ The assessment will allow you to determine which exercises are appropriate for you and your current level of conditioning.

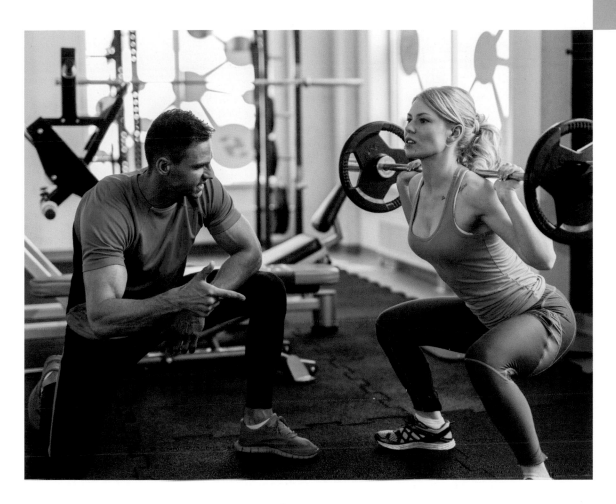

should be able to help you make an informed decision about whether it's appropriate for you to proceed. There are a lot of conditions and injuries for which the assessment and subsequent exercises would be extremely beneficial. For example, many riders find that a couple of hours into a ride they suffer from soreness or tightness in their lower backs. Assuming that their bike set-up is correct and they've no past or current underlying injury concerns that may be responsible, this book provides a systematic way to identify issues and address them with appropriate and beneficial exercises.

You need to be willing to commit to off the bike conditioning as a regular part of your training plan. To make progress, you have to dedicate time to it regularly and consistently. It's not a quick fix but, if followed correctly, will benefit you both on and off the bike for the rest of your life.

You don't need previous experience of off the bike conditioning or gym work. Full instructions, including photo demonstrations, are provided for all assessment tests and subsequent exercises. In fact, you're probably better off if you are starting with a blank slate as many riders who have dabbled with strength work in the past have ingrained bad habits, have received poor instruction or find it frustrating when their previous loads are reduced to correct faults in form.

You may also have been told by a coach, bike fitter or even a club mate that strength work would help you to overcome some issues that you have with your cycling. Unfortunately, such advice is rarely backed up with an appropriate routine. You'll either be given a generic routine or left to research one for yourself. With the assessment and exercises in this book, you'll know, right from the start, that you're performing exactly the right movements for your specific needs.

▼ *Even within the pro peloton, an exercise routine that works for one rider can be totally inappropriate for another.*

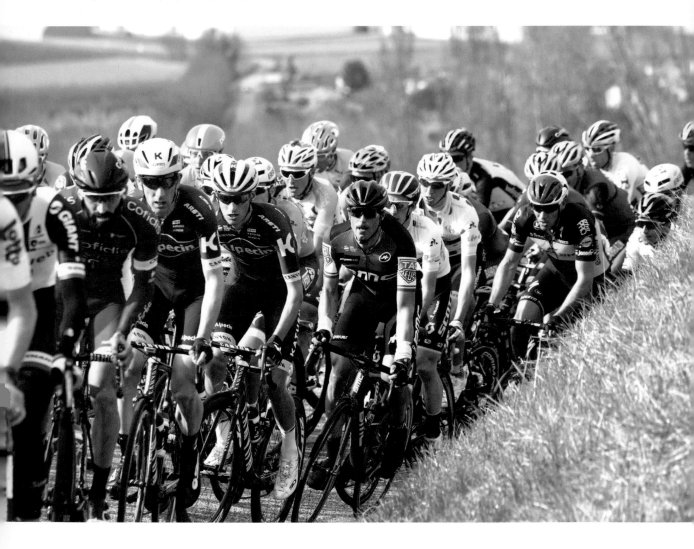

Degrees of freedom and range of movement (ROM)

Although we'll use the term 'degrees of freedom' a lot in this book, it may not be familiar to you. We'll use it instead of referring to flexibility, which can be confusing and misleading. Strictly speaking, the word flexibility refers to flexion, which is simply how much a joint can bend, and there is so much more to movement than this.

Another related term we'll use is range of movement (ROM). This is a measurement in degrees of how far a joint, say your knee, can move through. A physiotherapist can measure ROM with a tool known as a goniometer. A less mobile joint has a lower range of movement and therefore fewer degrees of range.

If someone wants to perform a complex multi-joint movement such as a squat correctly, they need good ROM at several joints – the ankles, knees and hips, for a start. If they have a few degrees of ROM missing in their ankles but good ROM at their knees and hips, we would describe them as having good degrees of freedom (range) to perform a squat as, to a certain extent, they can make up for the ankles' loss at the other joints. This is an incredible capability of the human body, being able to compensate for limitations or restrictions in one area and find a way to allow us to perform certain movements.

However, this ability to compensate is limited and if the ankles were more restricted and the ROM available in the knees and hips slightly decreased, performing a good squat becomes much harder and carries an increased risk of injury. The movement is restricted by poor ROM at more than one joint to a point where it simply

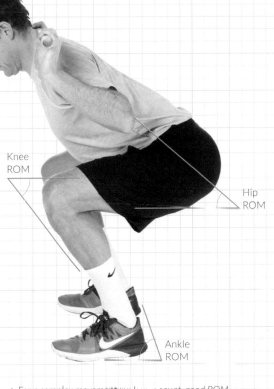

Knee ROM

Hip ROM

Ankle ROM

▲ *For a complex movement such as a squat, good ROM is required at a number of joints.*

cannot be performed well. We would therefore say that the degrees of freedom available to that individual to perform a squat are limited.

You can almost think of the ROM at each joint in your body contributing to an overall tally of degrees of freedom. By identifying and correcting limitations in ROM throughout your body, you'll up your tally – your degrees of freedom – for a range of movements, and your overall ability to move well.

HOW THE ASSESSMENT WORKS

There's a bewildering number of tests for almost every joint of your body but it's easy to get confused by information overload and many of the tests are difficult to self-conduct, so we've condensed things down to a few key body parts that commonly present problems for cyclists and are key during many lifting movements.

First, we examine movement around the hip area. We're starting here as this is the centre of your body, where many muscles attach. Having the necessary range and control of this area will dictate a lot of what goes on through the rest of your body. Staying with the trunk, we then look at the thoracic spine, assessing both rotation and extension. Moving up, we also assess the shoulders and, at the other extreme of the body, the ankle too. You might immediately question why we don't test the knee, but by testing both the lumbar spine/pelvis and the ankle we effectively do, as we look at two more complex joints above and below the knee. The relatively simple knee joint is a 'bad neighbour' as many of its problems are actually down to the joints above and below it. It's essential to think of the body as a whole and although we break it down, especially during the early stages of the assessment, you'll soon see how interrelated all the components are.

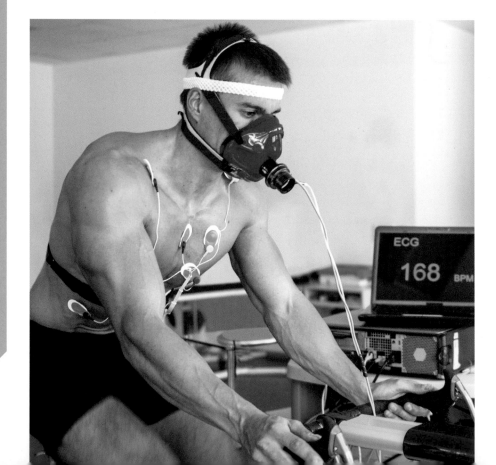

All of the tests can be conducted on your own but they are probably easier with the assistance of a partner, who'll be able to ensure you don't cheat and can maybe even film or photograph them for future reference. Work through each test in turn and if you fail to meet the standard set in any of them, you'll need to work on the exercises dedicated to resolving that issue before moving on to the next level. You can view it a bit like a game of Monopoly – fail a test, do not pass Go and go straight to exercise jail!

This doesn't mean, though, that you're in any way delaying benefitting your cycling. Simply by conducting the tests and identifying your areas of weakness, you're already progressing. By working on a continual cycle of test, train to those weaknesses and retest, you'll be building that broad base of conditioning. The assessment, and its accompanying exercises, will form the basis of your preparation routine before any off the bike conditioning session. You'll find that your levels will fluctuate significantly, even on a day-to-day basis. If you've done a hard ride, a long drive or put in some heavy work in the garden, you may find that tests you've previously passed are more of a challenge. It may just take a few minutes to work successfully on the area in question or you may find you have to revise your workout plans and priorities. For example, you might have planned to do a hard interval session on your time trial bike but find that, after a long day sitting on uncomfortable chairs in meetings, you feel tight around your hips and lower back. Rather than just ploughing on

with the session, you sensibly work through the assessment and discover your level is reduced compared with normal. You spend some time working on the movements that you know will help to correct the issue, reassess and find that you're back to an acceptable level. You can then do your intervals as planned, confident that your body is in a good place to deal with the demands of the session. If, however, you weren't able to mobilise the area successfully, it'd be better to change the session to some light spinning on the rollers followed by some dedicated mobilisation work and to move your time trial intervals to later in the week.

A great example of this from the Great Britain Cycling Team is Callum Skinner. Callum really struggles with the active straight leg raise (ASLR), one of the foundation movements in our assessment, and this has a direct bearing on his ability to effectively perform axially loaded exercises such as squats. If he tries loading these movements without addressing his ASLR, he develops problems with his lower back. For this reason, an ASLR test is an integral part of his pre-lifting routine and if he fails to reach the 75-degrees criterion, he has a number of exercises to try to improve it before moving on to his lifts. On some days he's able to sort it but on others, when he's unable to improve it, he has to reassess and adjust his training.

For many sportive and club riders, simply working until you complete the full assessment and are able to perform simple bodyweight strengthening exercises will have a significant positive impact on both your cycling and overall resilience. You'll have developed that broad base of conditioning and, unless you've specific performance goals such as time trialling or track cycling, maintaining that

◀ Testing your mobility and strength is as important as testing for your VO$_2$ Max or threshold.

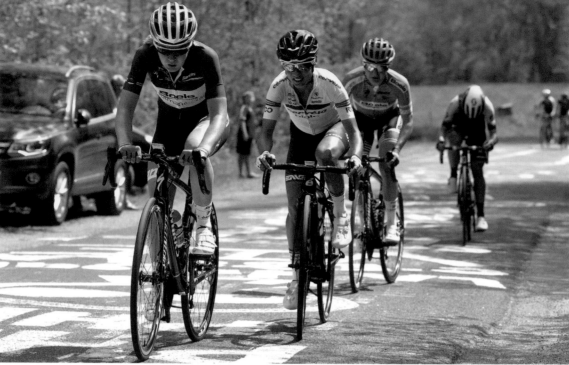

degree of conditioning would be a great attainable and maintainable goal.

The assessment looks at key areas of the body. These areas have been identified through our extensive experience working with cyclists and the common issues that they present with. Even riders who've succeeded at the highest level of the sport have these issues and it's only by putting in a lot of work that they can progress to loaded lifts in the gym. These riders are obviously strong on the bike but need a lot of input and effort to be able to conduct effective off the bike conditioning. For a few of the Women's Track Endurance Squad, being able to perform ten quality bodyweight squats represented a significant challenge. By examining these areas, we can guide you to the most effective exercises that will allow you to progress and target common sites for injury, which are often also where you'd benefit most from strengthening. You won't waste time working through a vast list of unnecessary

▲ *Even riders who've succeeded at the highest level of the sport have the sort of issues that the assessment will flag up.*

exercises that aren't applicable to you or are possibly unsuitable and even dangerous. When Phil first started working with Sir Bradley Wiggins, his professional team had given him a bewildering list of 27 exercises to be working on. He was rightly concerned about when he would find the time to actually ride his bike! This type of generic scattergun approach is typical of so many off the bike conditioning routines. By assessing and targeting your weaknesses, you can be sure you're doing the exercises that will be most beneficial for you. Three effective and targeted exercises done regularly and well are far better than a list of ten done haphazardly every now and then.

For these key areas of the body, we then assess at three levels before moving on to dedicated strength training.

Range of movement

There are numerous variables that can affect the ROM of a joint, including genetics, injury history and our daily lives. However, most limitations in ROM in adults come down to attrition and the wear and tear of life. If you take a baby or young child, most will display full ROM in the majority of their joints – look at how easily children can sit in a deep squat, displaying full ROM in their hips, knees, ankles and other key joints, and then compare this with the number of adults who can do this. Unfortunately, life is tough on our bodies. A torn hamstring that hasn't healed optimally will result in scar tissue that can easily limit ROM of both the hip and knee joints. Hours spent sitting at a desk, driving or even riding your bike can impact the ROM of numerous joints. Remember, the ROM of individual joints combines to give us degrees of freedom for any given movement involving these joints and if just one joint is compromised, the whole movement suffers. Fortunately, in most cases, you can do something about limited ROM, and while you might never be as good as your baby self, you can certainly be better than where you're currently at.

As a cyclist, you may question why we're looking for ROM beyond that required of a pedal stroke. The answer is resilience and that pyramid of conditioning. No matter how strong you were on the bike, your pyramid would be massively top heavy and hugely unstable. If your ROM at each of your joints is limited to what you'd experience on a bike, your degrees of freedom both on and off the bike will be extremely poor. On the bike, a slight change in position or a fatiguing muscle could lead to reduced performance, discomfort or even injury. Off the bike, you'd be a walking liability. Any movement that challenged you beyond this range, including many exercises and daily activities, would expose you to a high risk of injury.

Control through range supported

Once we've determined if you have sufficient ROM, we then need to see what control you have through it in a relatively simple and supported movement. Many people, some with genetically hyper-mobile joints, display exceptional ROM but have little control through that range.

There's a common misconception that people who lift heavy weights are big, bulky and 'muscle-bound'. However, Olympic weightlifters probably display some of the highest levels of control, through high levels of range and under extreme load, of any athletes. At the other end of the spectrum would be an untrained individual who, because of genetics, displays the same range of movement as an Olympic lifter. Although their body can achieve the same positions as the lifter, they have little control and certainly couldn't handle any loading in a safe manner.

Again using the example of an active straight leg raise, control is shown by being able to lower the leg from a 75-degree angle without faults occurring, such as the leg bending or the lower back leaving the floor. By bringing in the demand of control, more joints are involved and we move beyond a simple ROM test. However, because your bodyweight is supported in the active straight leg raise by lying prone on the floor, and the movement is effectively in one plane, it's not as demanding as a three-dimensional unsupported movement.

Control through range unsupported

This is a more complex movement involving higher levels of control and co-ordination across multiple joints and without support. This would include movements such as hip hinges, squats, split squats, press-ups and rows. The squat is a brilliant example as it requires range and control through a series of joints that must work together in order to maintain the integrity of the system. By being able to perform these movements using your bodyweight, you're in a position to be able to move on to loaded exercises, progressive structured training and dedicated strengthening work. For many riders, though, maintenance of this level would be an extremely beneficial and worthwhile goal.

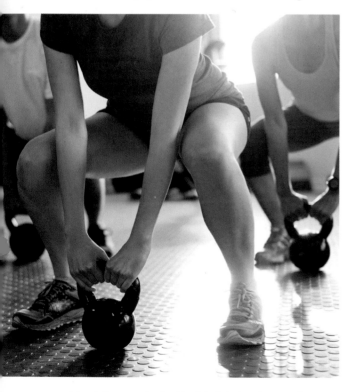

▲ *Loaded movements should only be introduced once you've worked successfully through the previous levels.*

Strength training

Once you have passed through the three levels of the assessment, if it fits with your cycling or other fitness and health goals you can move on to structured and loaded strength training. There will still be a progression of exercises to work through. For example, you will need to become proficient at goblet squats and other squat variations before moving on to more advanced loaded variations. Once you're at this stage of the programme, you will need to give careful consideration to how and when you incorporate lifting into your cycling training. We will go into detail on how to do this in Chapter 5. Remember, though, that you're not leaving the assessment and its associated movements behind – you will constantly revisit the assessment. Both riding and non-riding factors, such as a long drive or a heavy day in the garden, can cause regression, and you might also use it and its movements as part of your pre-lifting check and routine.

Assessment equipment

To be able to carry out the assessment, you will need some basic equipment.

- Dowel rod (or broomstick/PVC pipe)
- Protractor or goniometer
- Tape for marking wall and floor

For the more complex movements (hip hinge, squat, split squat, press-up and pull-up), it would also be beneficial to have a training partner to film you performing the test – using a mobile phone is fine. This will allow you to assess objectively how well you do.

Below are guidelines and images for the assessment movements. You should refer to the flow diagram and colour coding for the exercise prescriptions and priorities based on your performance. Be honest with yourself and don't be tempted to try to cheat the tests. It's not a bad thing or a reflection on your ability as a cyclist if you're unable to complete all or even any of the assessments. As we've already said, there are cyclists who have succeeded at the highest level of the sport who struggle with these tests or have had to put in a lot of work to be able to get through them.

Navigating the Flow Diagram

The flow diagram illustrates how you should work through the exercises in the book and devise the most appropriate and effective off the bike training routine for you.

It's strongly recommended that you read through the book and then come back to this flow diagram.

At the top of the flow diagram is range of movement (ROM) and the corresponding assessment movements. If you're able to complete these successfully, you would then move on to control through range supported and its assessment movements. If you fail to complete any of the range of movement assessments though, you would refer to the range of movement corrective exercises in Chapter 2. You would continue to work at this level, repeating the assessment movement, until you're able to progress.

Continue working through the flow diagram in this way, only moving on to the next level and set of exercises once you can complete the relevant assessment movement.

It should be noted that it is possible and likely that you'll be at different 'levels' for different body areas. For example, you could be working on control through range unsupported corrective exercises for your upper body but still be on range of movement corrective exercises for your lower body. Even within the lower body, you might be able to complete the active straight leg raise and lower but, due to a poor performance at the knee to wall assessment, you'd probably struggle with squats and split squats.

It's important to realise that your journey through the flow diagram won't be linear and, due to your training and other factors such as injury, you'll constantly fluctuate up and down the levels. However, you'll soon come to recognise your strengths and weaknesses and what areas you tend to need to work on.

ASSESSMENT MOVEMENTS

Assessment flow diagram

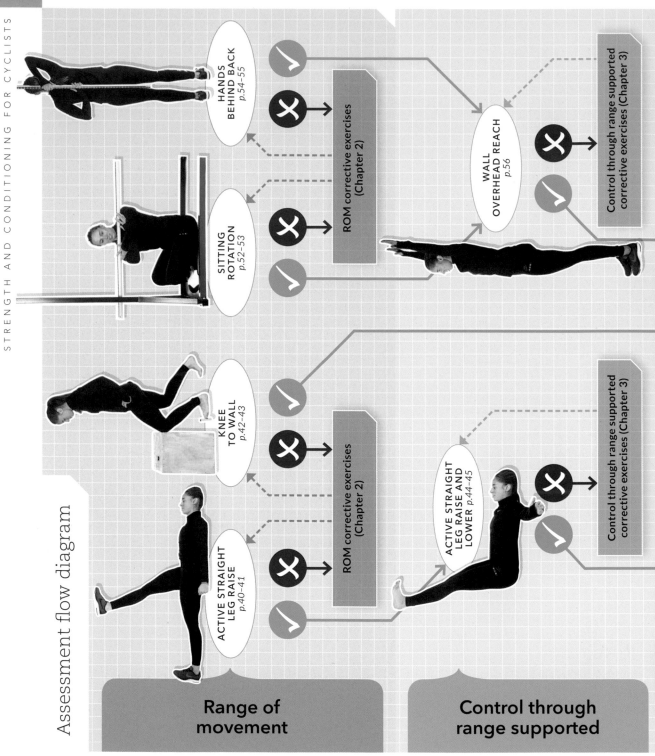

HANDS BEHIND BACK *p.54–55*

SITTING ROTATION *p.52–53*

KNEE TO WALL *p.42–43*

ACTIVE STRAIGHT LEG RAISE *p.40–41*

WALL OVERHEAD REACH *p.56*

ACTIVE STRAIGHT LEG RAISE AND LOWER *p.44–45*

ROM corrective exercises (Chapter 2)

ROM corrective exercises (Chapter 2)

Control through range supported corrective exercises (Chapter 3)

Control through range supported corrective exercises (Chapter 3)

Range of movement

Control through range supported

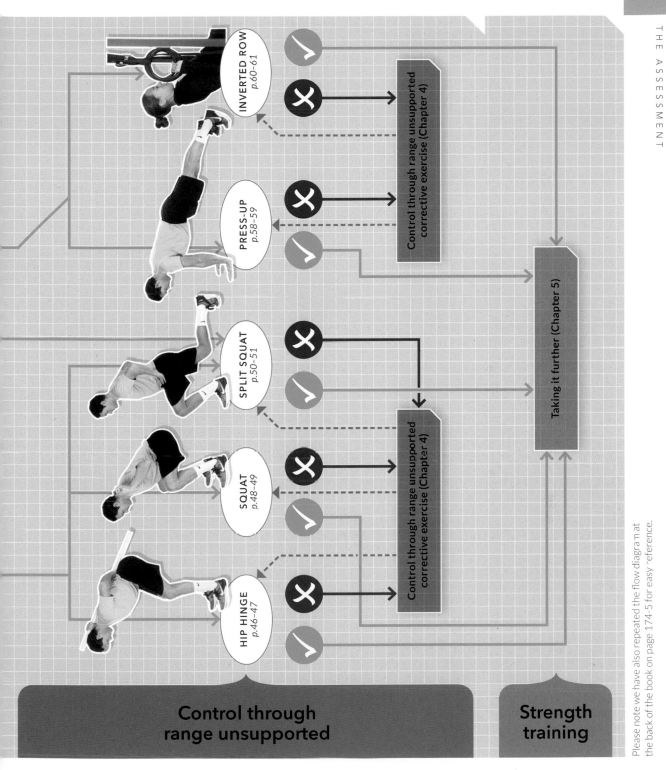

INVERTED ROW *p.60-61*

PRESS-UP *p.58-59*

SPLIT SQUAT *p.50-51*

SQUAT *p.48-49*

HIP HINGE *p.46-47*

Control through range unsupported corrective exercise (Chapter 4)

Control through range unsupported corrective exercise (Chapter 4)

Taking it further (Chapter 5)

Control through range unsupported

Strength training

Please note we have also repeated the flow diagram at the back of the book on page 174-5 for easy reference.

HIP, LUMBAR SPINE, PELVIS AND LEG

ROM: ACTIVE STRAIGHT LEG RAISE (ASLR)

GO: > 75 degrees
STOP: < 75 degrees or any other stop points

Superficially, the ASLR is a very simple test. However, do not be fooled by its simplicity as it can be very revealing. At first glance it may look like a test of hamstring flexibility and while it most certainly does assess that, it also highlights a number of other areas. It demands the ability to flex in one hip while the other leg is extended. As well as being linked to the action of cycling, this ability is key to all striding patterns such as walking, running and lunging. It shows up any differences, known as asymmetries, between your left and right side and assesses your ability to control your pelvis. You may even notice a stretching sensation in your calves during this test, showing that it's definitely not just about your hamstrings. By lying on the floor, your body is supported, which reduces the amount of control required to perform the movement. This makes assessing the ROM and performing the movement with the necessary strict form easier.

- Using a protractor and a metre rule, mark the point on the wall where a raise of 75 degrees would be.
- Lie on the floor on your back with your legs straight and together.
- Consciously push your lower back into the floor and maintain this contact throughout the test.
- Have your arms to your side at 45 degrees.
- Keep your toes up.
- Slowly raise one leg while keeping the other leg in contact with floor.
- A pass is successfully reaching 75 degrees without any of the fail points.
- Repeat with the other leg.

⚠ Stop points:

- Pain or cramping during the movement.
- Inability to maintain lower back contact with the floor.
- Inability to maintain non-lifting leg contact with the floor.
- Failure to maintain a toes-up foot position.
- Discrepancy between the legs.*
- Failure to reach 75 degrees.

*Any noticeable difference in ability between the legs may indicate an imbalance and should be viewed as a 'stop', especially if either leg fails to reach the 75-degrees target.

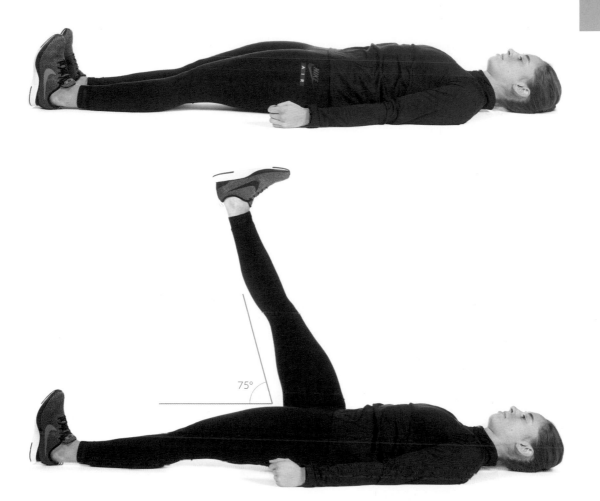

75°

▶ Even if you can reach
75 degrees, arching your
back is a stop point.

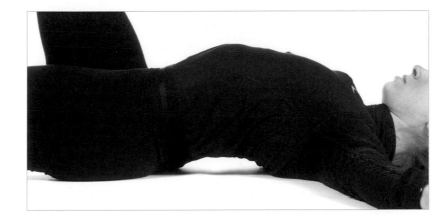

ROM: KNEE TO WALL

GO: > 11cm from wall
STOP: < 11cm from wall or any other stop points

Full ankle ROM is important as it is one of the key links in being able to perform more complex movements, such as squats. If your ankle is unable to dorsiflex sufficiently (the foot flexing up towards the shin), movements involving the joints above it, even if they have full ROM, will be compromised. As with all joints, it's a case of use it or lose it. If you don't regularly move a joint through its full range, the capacity of that range will decrease. Although there is a certain amount of 'ankling' during a pedal stroke, the movement is very small compared with what your ankle should be capable of. Incidentally, if you're a triathlete, poor ankle ROM, especially extension (pointing your toes), is a major limiting factor to an effective front crawl leg kick.

■ Make a mark on the floor 11cm away from the wall.
Stand facing the wall with your shoes off.
■ Put the big toe of one foot up to the mark and then attempt to bend the knee so it touches the wall.
■ Keep your hips square, but you can bend and adjust the position of the other leg to facilitate the movement.
■ Repeat with the other leg.

⚠ Stop points:

■ Pain or cramping during the movement.
■ Failure to reach the 11cm mark.
■ Discrepancy between the legs.

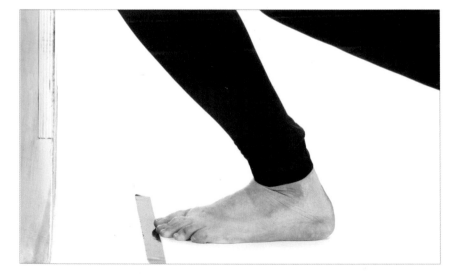

◄ *Set up a mark for your toes 11cm away from the wall.*

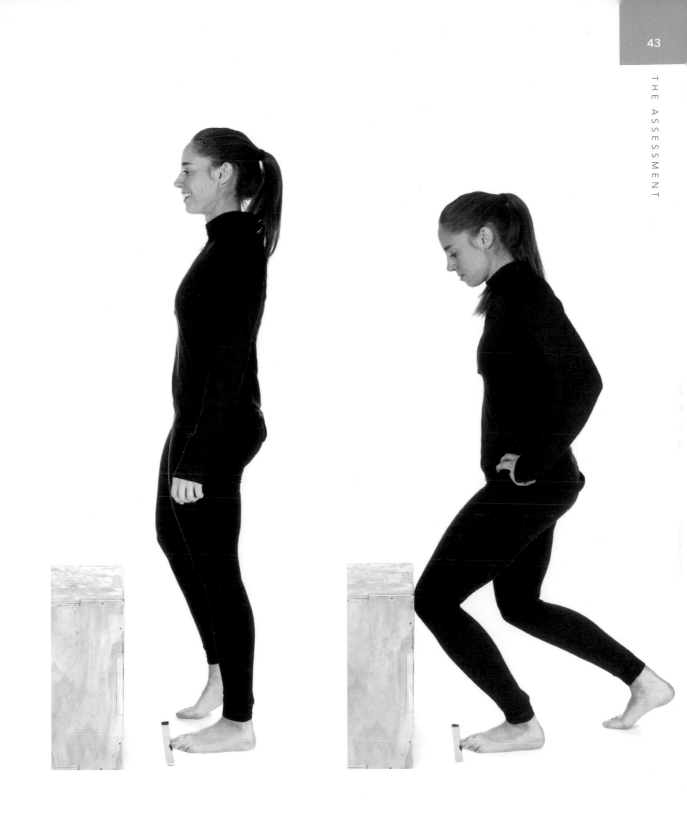

CONTROL THROUGH RANGE SUPPORTED: ACTIVE STRAIGHT LEG RAISE AND LOWER

GO: Full control throughout range with no cheat movements
STOP: Poor control and/or use of cheat movements or any other stop points

Once you've discovered from the active straight leg raise that you have sufficient range, you need to see what control you have through this range and, again, symmetry in both legs. As you progress towards more complex multi-joint movements and loaded exercises, this control becomes vitally important. For example, you may have sufficient hip range to achieve a deep squat but lack the control in your lower back and pelvis to safely load it. A good analogy of why control is so important is that you can't shoot a cannon off a canoe.

■ Successfully perform an active straight leg raise.
■ Take a breath at the top of the movement, exhale and lower the leg under control.
■ Repeat with the other leg.

⚠ Stop points:
■ Pain or cramping during the movement, especially in the hamstring.
■ Inability to maintain lower back contact with the floor.
■ Inability to maintain non-lifting leg contact with the floor.
■ Bending the knee during lowering.
■ Failure to maintain a toes-up foot position.
■ Holding your breath.
■ Discrepancy between the legs.

▶ *Be especially aware of maintaining lower back contact with the floor during the lowering phase.*

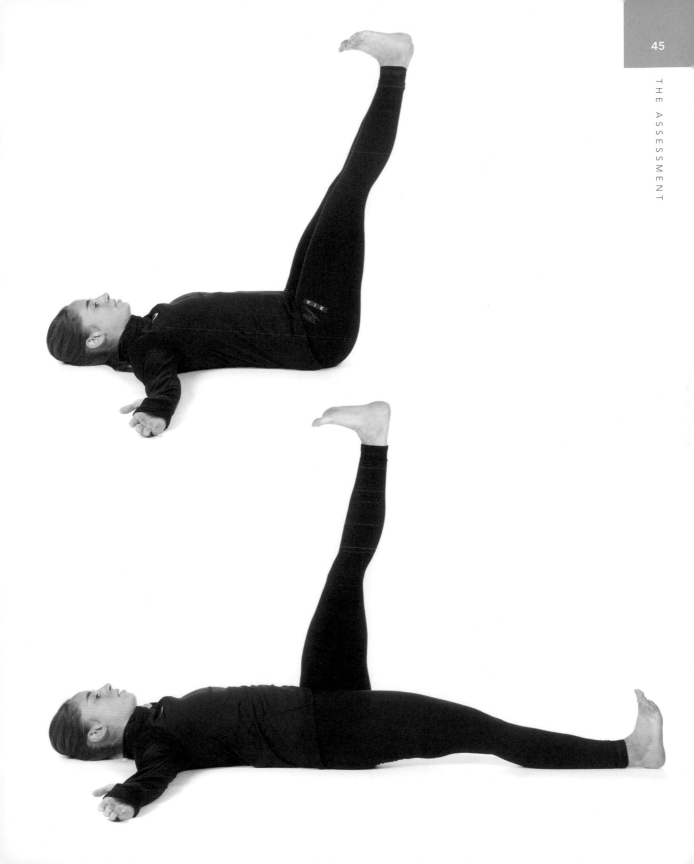

CONTROL THROUGH RANGE UNSUPPORTED: HIP HINGE

GO: Maintain contact points throughout movement
STOP: Lose any contact point or any other stop points

The hinge pattern is essentially the same action as an active straight leg raise and Lower; however, it reduces the amount of support involved, as you are no longer lying on the floor, and therefore increases the amount of control required. A hip hinge is a fundamental of human movement as it looks at your ability to shift your weight backwards while controlling the position of your spine and pelvis. Every time you bend forward at the hips, especially if picking something up, a correct

hip hinge, rather than rounding your back, is optimal. The ability to do this is crucial to sparing your spine and has been linked to avoiding back pain. In the gym, this movement is integral to movements such as the dead lift and also to certain squatting techniques. If this movement is performed incorrectly and then loaded, you're putting strains on your body that it's not designed for. A classic example of this is the number of athletes who report lower back discomfort after performing dead lifts. This has led to a commonly held misconception that dead lifts are bad for your back. However, the question to ask is, is it the exercise that's the problem or the way it's being performed?

▼ *If you struggle to hold your time trial position, off the bike work could definitely help.*

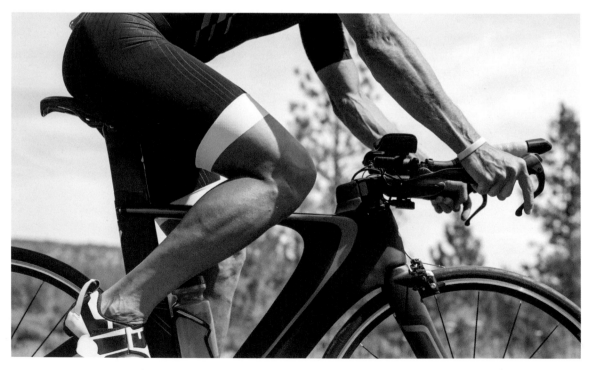

■ Using a protractor and a metre rule, mark a 50-degree angle on the wall.

■ Stand upright with your feet approximately shoulder-width apart and with straight but not locked knees.

■ Hold a dowel as shown in the image above. The key contact points that must be maintained throughout the test are: Dowel touching back of head, upper hand touching back of neck, dowel touching upper back, lower hand touching lower back and dowel touching tailbone.

■ Hinge by pushing your hips backwards. You can bend your knees slightly.

■ Aim for a torso angle of <50 degrees, pause and return to the start position.

■ As this movement is more complex, you may wish to get a friend to video it from side on to assess your form.

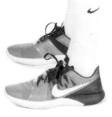

<50°

⚠ Stop points:

■ Pain or cramping during the movement.

■ Failure to reach a torso angle of 50 degrees.

■ Excessive bending of the knees. The aim is for straight but not locked.

■ Losing any of the contact points with the dowel at any stage of the movement.

CONTROL THROUGH RANGE UNSUPPORTED: SQUAT

GO: Be able to perform a deep squat
STOP: Any stop points

Squatting, like hinging, is a fundamental movement pattern. You only have to observe babies and young children to see how, for them, a squat is a comfortable and sustainable position. In developing countries, squatting is part of everyday life, not least for going to the toilet. It's only in the developed world, with our sedentary lifestyles involving hours spent seated at desks, driving or on the sofa, that we lose this ability and develop associated problems. There is a difference between the ability to deep squat compared with loaded squatting to enhance performance. For the purpose of the assessment we are looking at your ability to perform a deep squat, as this is a fairly good indicator of overall movement capability. A degree of lower back rounding is acceptable for the assessment but if you progress to loaded squats, this fault has to be eliminated. The later chapter on strength training will discuss squatting for performance enhancement in more detail.

The ability to get into a deep squat position is largely dependent on the degrees of freedom you have in your lower body but also significantly involves your upper body. Without good thoracic extension, you'll be unable to keep your torso parallel to your shins, which is crucial to good squatting. As a complex movement involving multiple joints, it's also dependent on your ability to be aware of your body in space and then coordinate it to perform the pattern. The ability to perform a deep squat is crucial to being able to perform loaded squat movements during strength training. If you're unable to perform a good unloaded deep squat and then add load, you're asking for trouble. You'll be loading near the limits of your ranges, which is a recipe for poor gains and potential injury. It's staggering how many cycling conditioning books prescribe barbell squats, a highly complex and demanding movement that's right at the apex of the squat hierarchy, without any attention being paid to whether the rider can perform them effectively and safely. From experience, even working with elite riders, most cyclists can't!

Torso not remaining parallel with shins

Knees going forward beyond your toes

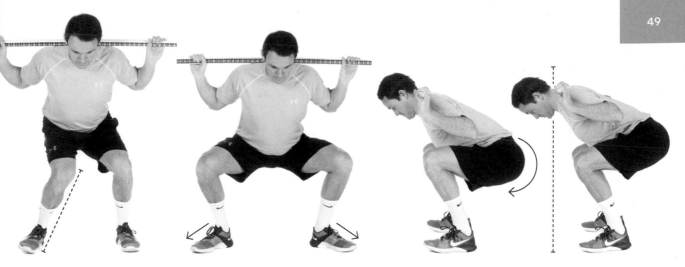

Knees collapsing in (valgus knee)

Feet rotating out into an excessive duck-footed stance

Pelvis tucking under your body (butt wink) and/or lumbar flexion

The dowel not remaining aligned over your feet

■ Place the dowel across the back of your shoulders. It shouldn't be resting on your neck but slightly lower down. Your hands should be gripping the dowel slightly wider than shoulder-width. If you find this position uncomfortable or difficult to achieve, you will probably also struggle with the hands behind back and wall overhead reach tests, and need to work on this area. If this is the case, you can perform the squat without the dowel.

■ Stand with your feet about shoulder-width apart and with your toes facing straight forwards or slightly outwards

■ Brace by engaging your glutes, pulling your ribcage down and tensing your trunk muscles.

■ Set your shoulders and upper body by pulling your shoulders back.

■ Start to lower by simultaneously hinging at the hips and bending your knees.

■ Keep your shins as vertical as possible, your head neutral, and drive your knees out to the side.

■ As you lower there will be a forward lean but your spine should remain neutral with minimal rounding, parallel to your shins, and the dowel should always be aligned over your feet.

■ You should aim to achieve a depth where your hips are below your knees and your thighs are below the horizontal.

■ Return to the start position, maintaining the form points above.

■ As this movement is more complex, you may wish to get a friend to video it from side on to assess your form.

⚠ Stop points:

■ Pain or cramping during the movement.

■ Inability to achieve a depth where your thighs are below the horizontal.

■ Your torso not remaining parallel with your shins.

■ Your knees going forward beyond your toes.

■ Your knees collapsing in (valgus knee).

■ Your feet rotating out into an excessive 'duck-footed' stance.

■ Your pelvis tucking under your body ('butt wink').

■ The dowel not remaining aligned over your feet.

CONTROL THROUGH RANGE
UNSUPPORTED: SPLIT SQUAT

GO: Be able to perform a split squat
on both sides
STOP: Any stop points

The third fundamental movement
pattern that we're assessing is the split
squat. It should be obvious, whether you're
walking, running or pedalling, that you do
so from an asymmetrical split stance. To
perform it successfully, you need optimal
degrees of freedom and control of both
legs in the opposing positions of hip
flexion and extension. The hip of the front
leg will be flexing and the hip of the rear
leg extended at the bottom of a split squat
or lunge. As with a squat, it requires
control of your spine and, because of the
split stance, a greater demand on your
balance and spatial awareness. Again, if
you start loading this movement – even if
it's only holding dumbbells or kettlebells
– before you can perform it well, you'll
be trying to strengthen a fundamentally
flawed system. It's a movement that's
really worth persevering with and getting
right, though. Variations of it are key
components of any good cycling strength
routine, and a rear foot elevated squat,
also known as a Bulgarian squat, for
example, is probably one of the best
exercises cyclists can do.

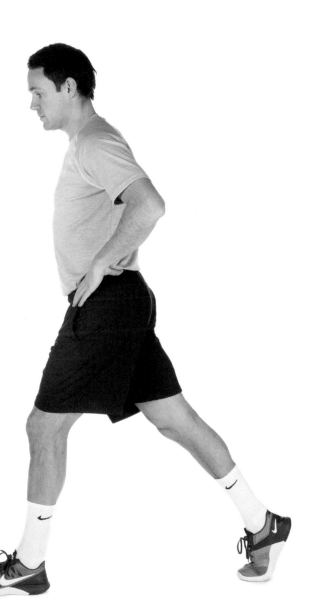

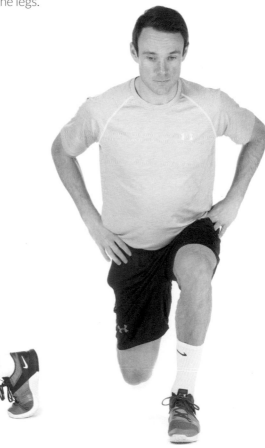

- From a standing position, take an exaggerated step forwards, keeping your feet in line or very slightly offset.
- As you do so, lift the heel of your rear foot and effectively perform a hip hinge. This creates a forward lean. A common coaching fault for split squats and lunges is to try to maintain an upright torso.
- Brace your trunk muscles and maintain a neutral spine.
- By bending both legs at the knees, drop towards the ground. Think of a straight-down movement.
- Keep your front shin vertical and your knee above the midpoint of your foot.
- You're looking to achieve a 90-degree angle in both your front and rear knee.
- Return to the start position, maintaining the form points above.

- Switch your lead leg and repeat.
- As this movement is more complex, you may wish to get a friend to video it from side on to assess your form.

⚠ Stop points:

- Pain or cramping during the movement.
- Inability to achieve a depth where a 90-degree angle is achieved in your front and rear knees.
- Your front knee going beyond the midpoint of the foot.
- Your front knee collapsing inwards or wandering outwards.
- Losing balance at any stage during the movement.
- Discrepancy between the legs.

THORACIC SPINE

ROM: SITTING ROTATION

GO: Be able to touch door frame with dowel on both sides while maintaining form and position
STOP: Inability to touch door frame on either side or any stop points

Although rotation of your torso during cycling is fairly minimal (there's some when climbing out of the saddle or when checking behind you), it's during everyday life that limitations in this movement can cause problems. Think about when you lift your shopping or child out of the car: you're bending and rotating with a load. Unless you have good range for this movement, attempting it in such uncontrolled scenarios can be an injury risk. Moreover, if you lack this range of movement, you will be unable to complete a large number of key strengthening

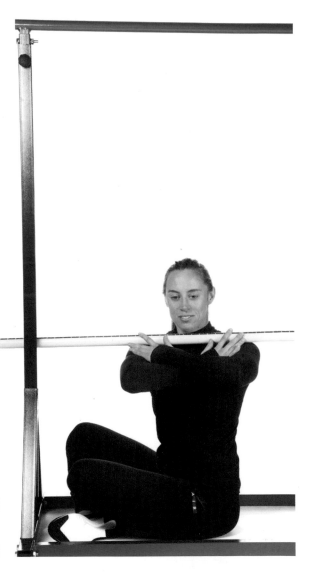

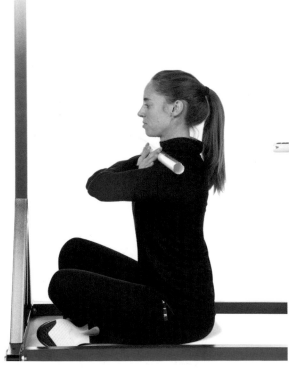

exercises as it is also a good indicator for thoracic extension. Thoracic extension is essential for many squatting and overhead movements. It's also a key parameter in achieving your most aerodynamic position on the bike.

■ Sit upright on the floor with your back straight, legs crossed and holding a dowel across your chest. Your knees should drop either side of the door frame.

■ Sit up tall and keep your head looking forwards.

■ Maintaining your arm and head position, rotate your torso.

■ Aim to touch the door frame in front of you with the dowel.

■ Repeat in both directions.

⚠ **Stop points:**

■ Failure to touch the door frame with the dowel.

■ Pain or cramping during the movement.

■ Discrepancy between sides (easier to rotate one way than the other).

■ The dowel does not remain level and in contact with the chest.

■ Inability to keep both buttocks on the floor.

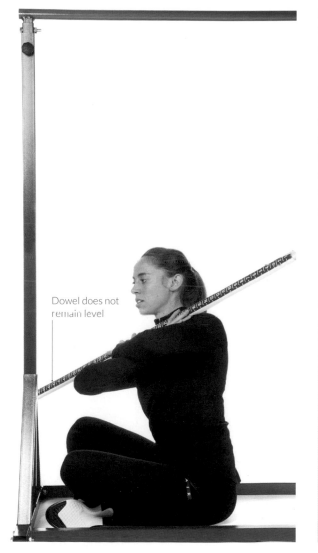

Dowel does not remain level

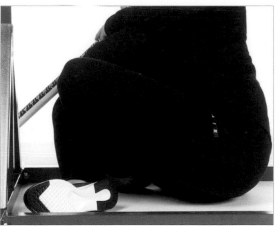

Inability to keep both buttocks on floor

ROM: HANDS BEHIND BACK

GO: Hands within 1½ fists' distance
STOP: Hands more than 1½ fists' distance or any stop points

A limitation in the range of motion in your shoulders can impact negatively on your cycling. Poor shoulder range can manifest as stiffness or pain in your shoulders and neck or an inability to sustain a more aggressive riding position on the drops. For time trial riders or track pursuiters, poor shoulder range can severely compromise your aerodynamic position. Even for many road riders, bringing their elbows closer together is one of the most effective ways of reducing frontal area and therefore drag. If your shoulders are stiff and unyielding, you're going to struggle to achieve and hold a good aero position. Shoulder limitations in range of movement will ultimately lead to more workload and stress being placed on other parts of the upper body, especially the neck and thoracic spine. It can also be a limitation to gym work as you'll struggle to hold a bar on your back during squats and find some pressing and pulling movements problematic.

■ Holding your dowel at the top, make a mark approximately 1½ fists' distance from the bottom of your hand.
■ Standing upright with your back straight and holding the dowel with one hand behind your head with the thumb of that hand downwards.
■ By lowering that hand and reaching upwards with the other behind your back, bring your hands as close together as possible. Avoid hitching your hands on the dowel and creeping them closer to each other.
■ When you've brought your hands as close together as possible, let go with the top hand and see if your bottom hand has reached the mark you made.

⚠ Stop points:
■ Failure to attain 1½ fists' distance between hands.
■ Hitching or creeping the hands closer together.
■ Pain or cramping during the movement or on release.
■ Excessive arching of the thoracic spine.
■ Discrepancy between sides.

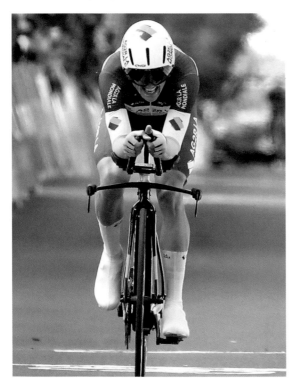

◄ *Bringing your elbows together is one of the most effective ways of reducing frontal area.*

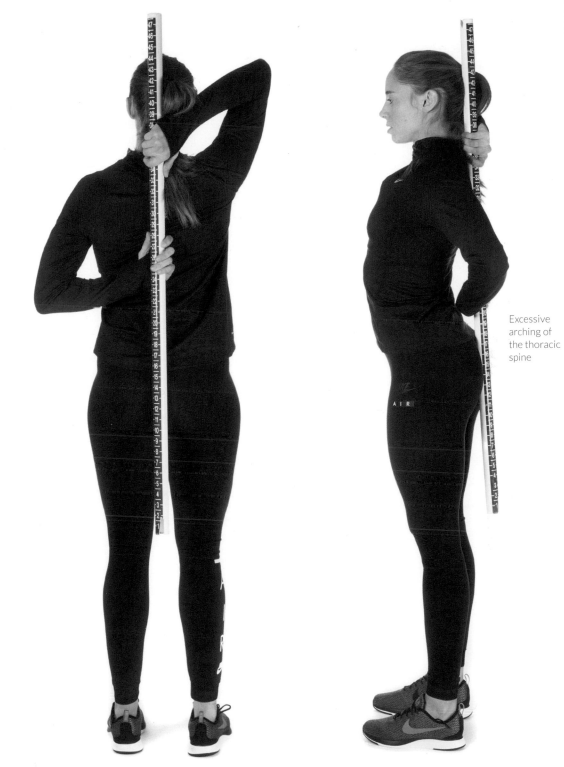

Excessive
arching of
the thoracic
spine

CONTROL THROUGH RANGE SUPPORTED: WALL OVERHEAD REACH

GO: Touch thumbs to wall
STOP: Inability to touch thumbs to wall or any stop points

This test looks at a number of key areas. It's another test of shoulder range; it assesses your ability to control your pelvis; and it looks at how well you can extend your thoracic area. All of these are vital to maintaining a strong and sustainable position on the bike, and good thoracic extension is key to being able to effectively perform movements such as the hip hinge and squat. This is a great example of how multiple areas of the body interact and are dependent on one another to perform complex movements. If one piece of the puzzle is missing, degrees of movement are limited and the movement is compromised. Finally, any overhead lift, whether a simple shoulder press or an advanced Olympic lift such as a snatch, requires full overhead range.

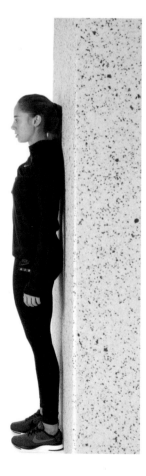
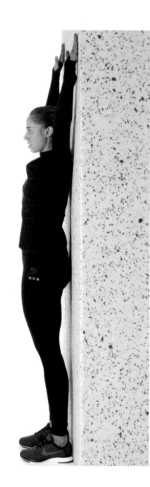
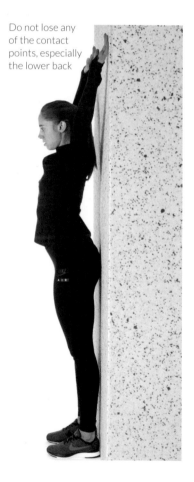

Do not lose any of the contact points, especially the lower back

Nature versus nurture

As with most aspects of sports performance, the way you're able to move is down to a combination of your genetics and your lifestyle factors. There's a fair amount of truth in the statement that you're born an Olympic champion, but between birth and the podium a lot of other factors have to click and a lot of hard work has to be done. You can't change bad genetics but there's a lot that can be done to improve the hand your parents dealt you. We've already talked about the work that Ben Swift puts in off the bike to improve his resilience, robustness and performance. Co-author of this book Martin Evans has a condition known as a cam hip impingement. This occurs when the ball-shaped end of the femur is not perfectly round. This interferes with the femoral head's ability to move smoothly within the socket. However, with much work on strength and mobility around the hip,

Martin is able to safely perform most exercises and movements. At the other end of the scale are people who are lucky enough to be born with excellent movement. In the Great Britain Cycling Team, Jason Kenny is the stand-out example of an athlete who's incredibly genetically blessed regarding his movement patterns. However, it's very easy to ruin good genetics. Modern life, especially the amount of time we spend seated in a hunched-over flexed position (including time spent on the bike), can compromise even the most genetically blessed individual. Nature does also tend to give and take in equal measure. For example, if you have a proportionally long back and short legs, you should be able to achieve a very aerodynamic time trialling position. However, the downside of this body shape is that, due to the length of your spine, you'd be more prone to lower back issues and would probably have to work hard on your ability to control movement patterns such as squats.

- Standing facing away from a wall, have your feet about shoulder-width apart and your heels close to the wall. Experiment with the distance that feels right to you.
- Lean back against the wall and make contact with your buttocks, lower back, shoulder blades and the back of your head.
- Turn your arms so that your thumbs are facing forwards.
- Keeping your arms straight, thumbs up and maintaining all contact points, slowly raise your arms above your head.
- Aim to touch the wall above your head with your thumbs and then lower.

⚠ **Stop points:**
- Failure to touch the wall with your thumbs
- Bending your arms.
- Changing your hand position.
- Losing any of the contact points, especially the lower back.
- Pain or cramping during the movement or on release.
- Discrepancy between sides.

CONTROL THROUGH RANGE
UNSUPPORTED: PRESS-UP

GO: Perform a press-up
STOP: Fail to perform a press-up,
or any stop points

Go to almost any circuit or boot-camp-style workout class and you can guarantee that, at some point, you'll be doing press-ups. Unfortunately, you can also guarantee, especially as the participants are driven by the instructor or drive themselves to push out 'one more rep', that they'll be done badly. A properly performed press-up, though, is a brilliant exercise and a great demonstration of upper body range and stability. It's a precursor to all the more advanced pressing movements, such as bench presses and dips. Although cyclists don't require huge levels of upper body strength, developing some will aid long climbs out of the saddle and bracing against the force of a sprint effort, and make you more resilient in day-to-day life.

Inability to keep elbows in line with hands

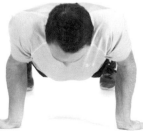

Hands rotating outwards (fingers not pointing straight forwards)

Modified press-ups

Some riders, although they may be able to set themselves up for a full press-up, lack the upper body strength to complete the full movement. In this test, we're not assessing strength so it can be appropriate to use a modified version of the movement. One solution that's often presented is to drop to your knees, but this isn't ideal for a number of reasons. Firstly, it can cause you to shift your whole body backwards, moving your shoulders behind your hands and putting an unnecessary strain on them. Secondly, it's discouraging the development of an optimal whole body stabilisation pattern. Finally, it's a short-term 'cheat' rather than a progressive modification. The solution is to elevate your hand position by performing the press-up on a bench or step. This allows you to work through the full movement but effectively reduces the weight you have to lift.

■ Kneel down with your hands shoulder-width apart and your fingers pointing straight ahead.
■ Lift your knees off the floor, have your feet and knees together and actively squeeze your glutes. Make sure your shoulders are directly above your hands.
■ Begin to lower yourself by bending your elbows. Keep your forearms vertical and your elbows in line with your wrists. Don't let your elbows flare out or allow your shoulder blades to come together.
■ Think about stiffening your whole body by clenching the buttocks and bracing the stomach. There should be a straight line from the back of your shoulders to your heels without any arching or sagging.
■ Full depth is a position where your chest is a fist's height off the floor.
■ Push back up to the set-up position, maintaining form and position.

⚠ **Stop points:**
■ Failure to perform a press-up.
■ Inability to reach full depth.
■ Inability to keep your elbows in line with your hands.
■ Your hands rotating outwards (fingers not pointing straight forwards).
■ Arching or sagging of the back.

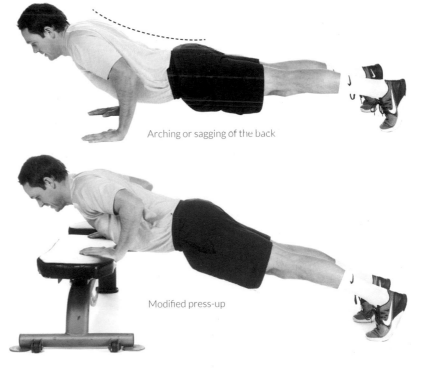

Arching or sagging of the back

Modified press-up

CONTROL THROUGH RANGE UNSUPPORTED (OPTIONAL): INVERTED ROW

GO: Perform an inverted row
STOP: Fail to perform an inverted row or any stop points

This assessment is optional as you may not have the necessary rings or suspension training system to be able to perform it. It's effectively an inverted press-up, looking at a very similar movement pattern but through a pulling rather than a pushing motion. If you're climbing out of the saddle or sprinting on your bike, each side of your upper body is effectively alternating between pushing and pulling. Because of the amount of time we spend in a flexed forward position, on your bike and at a desk, working on pulling movements can help strengthen the upper back muscles that are critical to maintaining good alignment through the shoulder joint.

- Set the height of the rings according to your strength/ability. The closer your body is to being parallel to the floor, the harder it will be.
- The rings should be shoulder-width apart and you should grip them with your palms facing in.
- With your heels remaining on the floor, adopt an 'inverted press-up' position. All the same cues apply. Keep your shoulders, elbows and wrists in line, engage your glutes, brace and maintain a straight line from the back of your shoulders to your heels.
- Keep your elbows and wrists in line and, without arching or sagging, pull your chest towards your hands. Avoid 'turtling' your shoulders up towards your ears.

- Full range is when your wrists come level with the top of your chest.
- Lower back to the start position under control, maintaining form and position.

⚠ Stop points:
- Failure to perform an inverted row.
- Inability to reach full range.
- Inability to keep your elbows in line with your hands.
- Arching or sagging of the back.

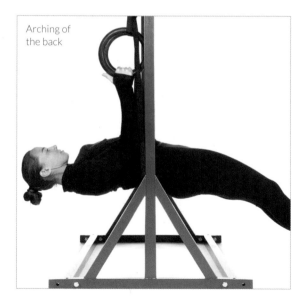

Arching of the back

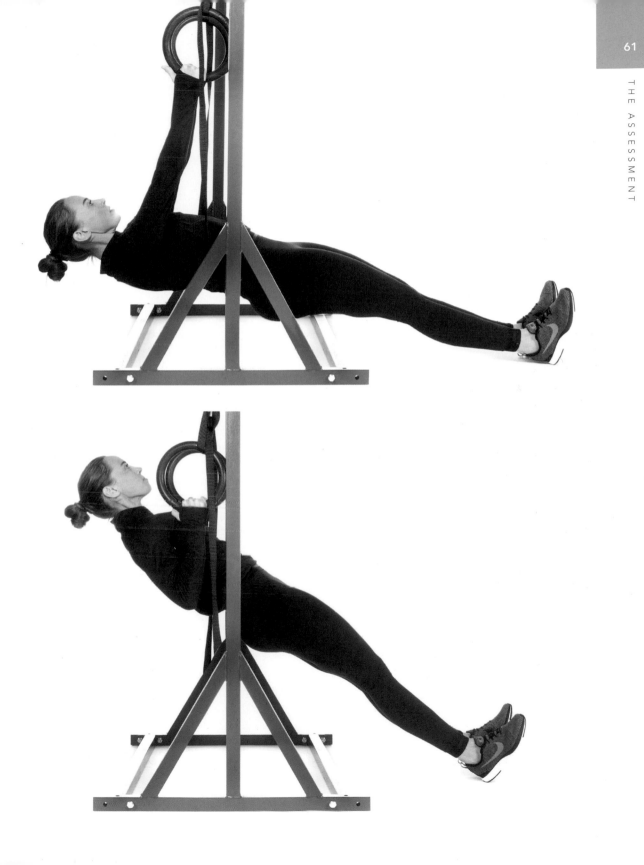

CHAPTER SUMMARY

Until you assess, you've no idea what issues you have

The majority of cycling training manuals prescribe generic strength and off the bike conditioning routines with no consideration given to the individual needs of the athlete. This can result in time wasted through unnecessary and ineffective exercises, and, if the exercises are not suited to the rider's current physical qualities and movement capabilities, potential injury.

View the assessment as part of your training

The temptation for many riders, especially if they have some previous strength training experience, is just to go straight to the gym, load up a leg press or squat bar and start hammering out the three sets of ten reps they've always done. They probably view the assessment and the limitations it potentially puts on their training as an unnecessary obstruction to their progress. This couldn't be further from the truth, and the rider described above would probably gain massively from working through the assessment and subsequent exercises. From the first time you attempt and assess your active straight leg raise, you'll be starting on a bespoke journey towards greater resilience and cycling performance.

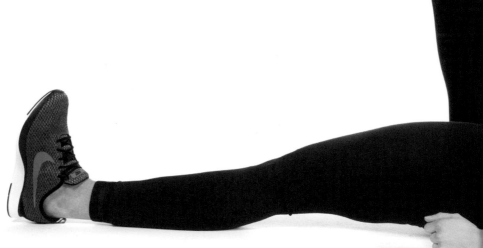

Don't see fails as failures

We deliberated and fretted as to how to describe the stop points in the assessment and whether using the word 'failure' seemed too negative. However, the percentage of cyclists, even at the highest level of the sport, who would consistently pass every test is minuscule. As we've already described, there are Olympic champions who have to work daily on specific movements to be able to then move on to their specific training. A fail in any of the tests is just an indicator of an area that needs work and, by addressing it, you can achieve significant improvement.

Find a friend

Although the majority of tests in the assessment can be performed individually, roping in a partner, who can also ideally video the movements, makes it far easier and more objective, and means you're less likely to cheat, whether intentionally or not. It can also be useful motivationally to have someone to work with.

Assess, reassess and repeat

The assessment isn't a one-off; you will constantly revisit it as you progress and move through your cycling year. You might find that at the end of your season, when maybe you hadn't been focusing on off the bike training so much, you have slightly regressed. One especially hard ride or a day of hard gardening can easily affect your performance and, by performing tests from the assessment, you can discover what training is appropriate for you at the moment.

The assessment and the tests in it are some of the most powerful and effective training tools at your disposal. They give you a snapshot of your body, its current state and the training you should (and, more importantly, shouldn't) be doing.

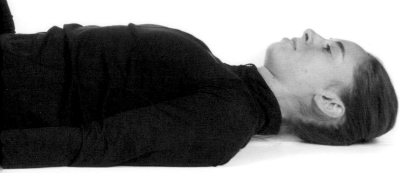

◄ *The assessment is at the heart of your off the bike training and you'll constantly revisit it.*

ROM CORRECTIVE EXERCISES

Once you have completed the assessment you will have discovered the areas of the body that need work. If you have failed any of the tests, there are a number of exercises described that you can use to correct that particular issue.

The exercises are listed in hierarchical order but as the exact cause of each issue will vary significantly from one rider to the next, you'll have to experiment to find the exercises and sequences that work best for you. The exercises and the order in which they are presented is based on our experience of working with elite-level cyclists and what usually limits them.

All of the body areas we're working on are extremely complex, with many muscles and other tissues attached. They interact and impact on one another, so there's no quick fix or single guaranteed 'magic bullet' exercise that will work for everyone. You should work through the suggested exercises in order and find which, for you, has the greatest effect by retesting the area you're working on. Once you have attained a pass in a particular test in the assessment, you can move on to the next level. This could take just one focused session or, for some issues and riders, significantly more consistent work over multiple sessions.

By working methodically through the assessment and the corrective exercises, you'll soon discover your personal issues and the most effective

exercises for resolving them. Determining which exercises these are could be as tangible as a resulting measurable improvement in the assessment or it could just be an exercise that feels right to you. Once you have discovered your key exercises, you can create bespoke routines that are tailored to your needs and time availability. If you're short of time or want to do bite-sized chunks of work daily, multiple times per day or pre/post ride, focus on a few key exercises. If you're looking to perform dedicated off the bike sessions and have more time to spare, simply increase the number of exercises you include.

The corrective exercises comprise two parts: tool-assisted self manual therapy (TASMT) and stretching.

▶ *A foam roller is an essential weapon in your off the bike training armoury.*

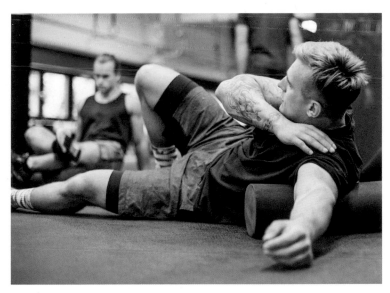

1. TOOL-ASSISTED SELF MANUAL THERAPY (TASMT)

TASMT uses a tool such as a foam roller, trigger point ball or peanut (effectively two trigger point balls joined together) to apply pressure and work on tight or restricted areas.

GENERAL GUIDELINES FOR TASMT

1 Explore the muscle you're working on for tight or restricted parts and spend time focusing on it. Don't just mindlessly roll back and forth.
2 Spend some time oscillating over and deep breathing on the restricted part.
3 Spend at least 2 minutes on the muscle group you're focusing on.
4 It needs to be done daily, ideally multiple times each day. Little and often, consistently, is the best approach.
5 It can be done any time during the day.

a) Pre-workout is particularly useful if you feel restricted or tight in an area, such as in your hamstrings after a long drive to an event, and it has been shown to increase flexibility acutely. However, avoid heavy or prolonged rolling immediately prior to training or racing.
b) Post-workout, there is some evidence that it can reduce delayed onset muscle soreness (DOMS).

It is recommended that the TASMT exercises are trialled first in the order listed. After performing the exercise as described, retest to assess if it has made a difference. After trialling the exercises in Stage 1, move on to the stretching movements of Stage 2 and repeat the same process.

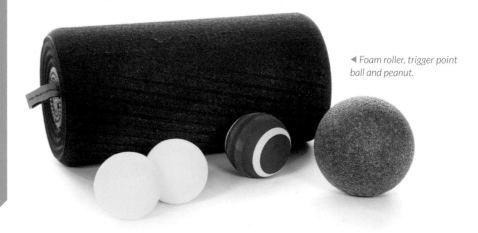

◀ Foam roller, trigger point ball and peanut.

The fascial release debate

Despite foam rollers being a staple in the kitbag of the majority of elite athletes, their use and effectiveness is still a matter of huge debate and controversy. The fasciae comprise a spider's-web-like network of white connective tissue that surrounds all of your muscles. All fasciae are connected and it can almost be thought of as a skinsuit surrounding our muscles. In a healthy state, the fascia is soft, flexible and free-moving, but repetitive movement, load and trauma can cause it to become tight and unyielding. As the name suggests, fascial release techniques, such as using a foam roller or trigger point ball, purportedly release the tissue and maintain it in a healthy, pliable state. The classic and most commonly rolled body part is the iliotibial band or ITB. Running down the length of your outer thigh from hip to knee, we tackle the muscles that attach and intertwine with it during the various 'smash' exercises we prescribe.

Some 'fascial release sceptics' would argue that as the ITB is an inert tendon (fascial) type structure, using a foam roller on it would have no physical effect or therapeutic benefit at all, while at the other end of the spectrum are 'fascial evangelists' who overindulge in a detailed description of the multi-layered world of fascia, how it is everywhere throughout our bodies and is the key to all problems. As with many things in life, the truth is probably somewhere in the middle of these extreme viewpoints. Fasciae are found throughout your body and are undoubtedly important but we'd probably have to double the word count of this book to explore all the relevant literature and that's certainly not going to help you to ride your bike faster. There are plenty of studies and articles that explore this debate further but, be warned, it's an ever-changing and polarising field with passionate experts in both camps.

What we can say, with over 20 years of sports medicine and training experience, is that foam rolling and other fascial release techniques work far more often than they don't. As with many areas, including medical interventions, training and nutrition, individual responses vary but our experience is that the overwhelming response of athletes to fascial release is positive.

We can't give you conclusive and indisputable reasons as to why it works, but it's probably down to a combination of factors including fascial manipulation, pain modification and muscular release. Returning to the example of foam rolling the ITB, from a fascial manipulation perspective, rolling probably alters the water content of the tissue, which we know is key to it functioning optimally. It's often a painful experience to inflict on yourself and so can modify the perceived level of pain overall. It's debatable as to whether the ITB has contractile elements so the input of a muscular release component is less clear. However, it integrates and connects with a huge number of muscles, some of which will be affected in a knock-on manner by the foam rolling.

In summary, in our experience of working with athletes, foam rolling and other fascial release techniques are beneficial. The hows and whys might not be 100 per cent clear or understood but we're not aware of a more effective self-massage and therapy technique for the loosening and release of soft tissue and it certainly doesn't do any harm. Heated debate around this topic will undoubtedly continue but we're confident in the benefit of these techniques and their place in your off the bike conditioning routine.

2. STRETCHING

Stretching looks to develop the comfortable range of movement of a muscle and, in combination with tool assisted self manual therapy (TASMT) form the cornerstones of the corrective exercises in this book. Many riders have a vague notion about stretching and might sporadically do a token bit but, to be effective, it has to be focused and done correctly.

GENERAL GUIDELINES FOR STRETCHING

1 Explore the muscle you're working on for tight or restricted parts; don't just hold a passive stretch (see box on page 70-71).

2 When you find a tight or restricted part, work through it by increasing and relaxing the intensity of the stretch. Breathe deeply as you do this.

3 If you struggle to maintain a consistent pattern of deep breathing, you have pushed the stretch too hard. Back off the stretch slightly, re-establish your breathing pattern and continue to develop the stretch.

4 Spend at least 2 minutes working on a specific stretch or muscle group.

5 Stretching needs to be done daily, ideally multiple times per day. Get out of the mindset that stretching has to be performed post-workout when your muscles are warm – it can be effective at any time. If you're sitting in front of the TV, do some stretching.

6 Some of the stretches give 'banded' options. The use of an elastic resistance band can enhance the stretch as it allows for the joint to be placed in its optimal position.

7 If performing pre-workout or competition, use the shorter duration, i.e. less than 45 seconds, as longer-duration stretching has been shown to acutely reduce strength and power production.

▶ *Focus on hydration and your recovery routine post-ride; leave stretching until you can focus on it properly.*

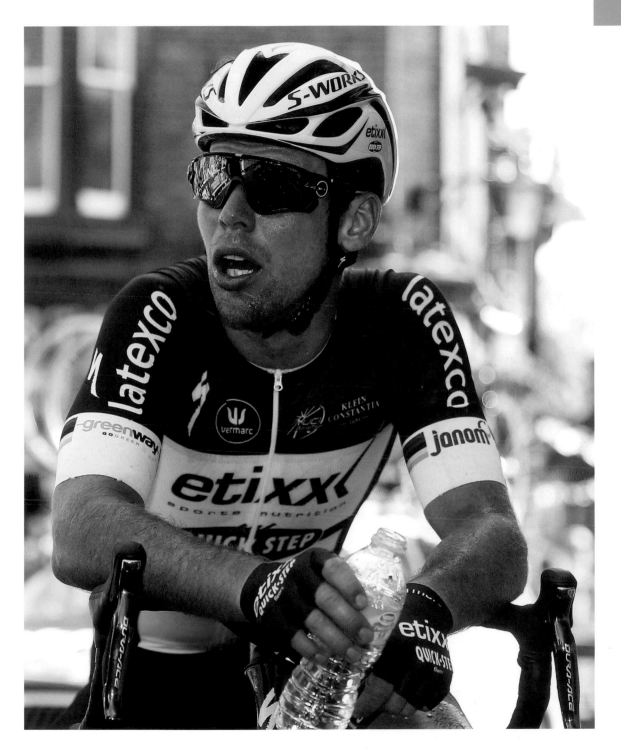

Stretching doesn't stretch

If you look up a definition of stretching, you'll find reference to applying force to an object to make it longer. However, when applied to the act of 'stretching' muscles, this isn't really the case. Muscles, due to their physical structure and having fixed points of origin and insertion, *can't become physically longer to an observable degree or to explain the benefits associated with stretching.* When we refer to a muscle being 'tight' it's because, for a number of reasons, it has become restricted and its range of motion is limited – but it *hasn't actually become shorter.* If you took an athlete with tight hamstrings and performed an active straight leg raise test, pain would prevent them from reaching full range. However, if you did the same test on the athlete under anaesthetic, you'd be able to force their leg to full range. If you broke your arm and it was plastered in a bent position for a month, when the plaster was removed you'd struggle to straighten your arm. This is because your biceps, which are 'stretched' when your arm is straightened, never attained full range while your arm was in plaster. The muscles haven't shortened during that time, they just need re-educating to allow a full range of motion. Muscle has a memory of what it has done recently and, if you push it beyond this, it'll resist, giving you discomfort or pain as a warning sign.

So, if you embark on a focused stretching regime, how can those gains in range of motion be accounted for if the muscle isn't becoming longer? The current consensus is that it's predominately down to how you perceive the sensation of stretching and how that perception can change. By constantly pushing your muscles to and slightly beyond the point where they tell you to stop, their sensory end point increases and they allow progressively more range.

In light of the above, although we'll refer to some exercises under the umbrella term of stretching, it's really a gross oversimplification and arguably inaccurate. When we talk about stretching, it can be helpful to think of three main types. Firstly, there are

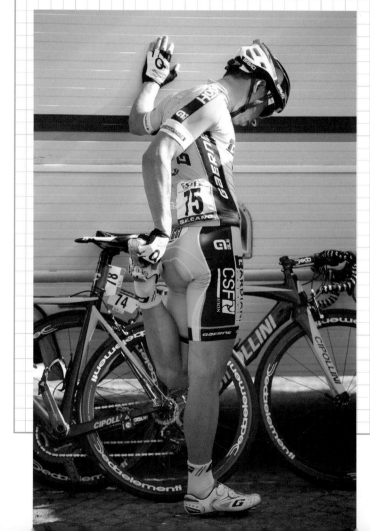

◀ *Unstructured stretching pre or post riding are unlikely to have any beneficial effect and can even negatively impact on performance.*

'ballistic' stretches. These are rapid movements that are often employed before activities and sports to work the athlete dynamically through the ranges of motion they're likely to employ. An example might be a scrum half in rugby going through a series of lunge-type movements. However, these types of stretches have little relevance for cyclists. Next are 'passive' stretches, where you assume a position to create a stretch on a muscle and hold it there using either another part of your body, some apparatus or the help of a partner. An example would be placing your leg on top of a table to create a stretch in your hamstring.

Finally, and what we'll mostly be prescribing, are 'active' stretches. In an active stretch, you utilise the fact that muscle groups work in pairs, an agonist and antagonist, and actively contract one to create a stretch on the other. An example would be during a rear foot elevated or Bulgarian squat. By engaging your glutes, you extend the hip and, in doing so, create a stretch on your quads.

'Active' stretch: rear foot elevated squat

'Passive' quad stretch

HIP, LUMBAR SPINE, PELVIS AND LEG

ROM: ACTIVE STRAIGHT LEG RAISE (ASLR) CORRECTIVES

Quad smash with foam roller

Cycling demands a lot of work from your quads but it's equally the time we spend seated at our desks and driving that contributes most significantly to problems with these muscle groups. In cyclists, this muscle group is the most likely culprit for the inability to achieve a satisfactory ASLR.

■ Adopt a plank position over the foam roller with your bodyweight supported by your elbows, forearms and toes.
■ With the roller positioned mid-thighs, lower yourself so that the majority of your weight is on the roller.

■ Rotate to one side to focus your weight on the leg you want to work on.
■ Bend the knee of the working leg and, by slowly rolling back and forth and rotating your body further to cover the outside areas of your thigh, seek out tight spots.
■ When you find a spot, oscillate on and off it for about 30–45 seconds or until you feel it release.
■ Find another tight spot and repeat this process, covering the whole thigh before moving on to your other leg.
■ You'll typically find you need to focus more on the outside of the muscle.

Tool-assisted self manual therapy (TASMT)

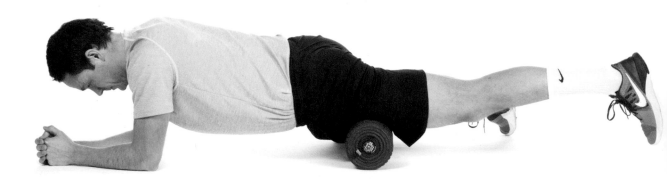

Hamstring smash with foam roller

Cyclists often present with tight or restricted hamstrings because cycling is a closed activity where you are locked in a fixed movement pattern and the knee doesn't typically extend beyond 35 degrees at the bottom of the pedal stroke. As we've already discussed, if a muscle isn't regularly taken through its full range (in the case of the hamstring, a fully straightened leg), it will become restricted. As well as creating possible problems off the bike when full extension of the leg is required, tight hamstrings can also negatively affect your riding. Tight hamstrings can be a contributing factor to lower back pain and, as they limit your ability to rotate your pelvis forwards, force you to flex entirely from your lower back and spine. This can compromise your ability to attain and hold an aerodynamic position. This is of particular relevance to time triallists and triathletes.

Tool-assisted self manual therapy (TASMT)

■ Start in a seated position with your hands directly under your shoulders and the roller positioned under the backs of your knees.

■ Bend the knee of the leg you're not working on and shift the majority of your bodyweight on to the leg still on the roller.

■ Roll back and forth to mid-thigh and look for areas of tightness. Rotate your foot outwards to focus on your outer thigh and inwards to concentrate on the inner.

■ If you find a tight spot, oscillate on and off it for about 30–45 seconds or until you feel it release.

■ Shift your start position so that the roller is now positioned mid-thigh. Repeat the process above but now working on the top half of your hamstrings up to your buttocks.

■ Repeat the whole process on your other leg.

■ You'll typically find you need to focus more on the outside of the muscle.

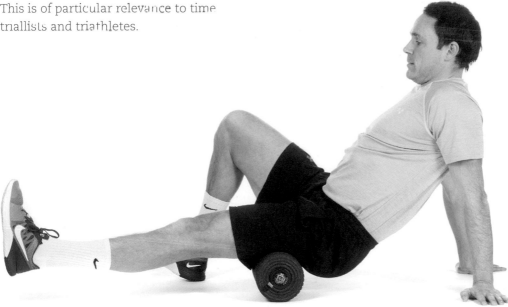

Glute smash
with foam roller

Along with the quads and hamstrings, the gluteal muscle group is also highly likely to be responsible for limiting ASLR performance in cyclists. This muscle group comprises the whole of your buttocks and is one of the most powerful in the body. They generate power and thrust in most movements, including running and cycling, by extending the hip. If restricted in their range, you'll be missing out on some of this power and your ability to rotate your pelvis on the hip will be limited. Not only will this prevent you from achieving a good ASLR right from the start of the movement, but, as discussed earlier, could also prevent you from achieving an aerodynamic riding position.

■ Sit on the foam roller with your legs bent and your hands directly below your shoulders.

■ Rotate on to the buttock that you want to work on and, to intensify the movement, cross the leg of the opposite side over your thigh.

■ Roll back and forth, changing the amount you rotate your body, to explore the whole buttock for areas of tightness or restriction.

■ If you find a tight spot, oscillate on and off it for about 30–45 seconds or until you feel it release.

■ Repeat for the other buttock.

■ You can use a trigger point ball for a more intense and focused version of this exercise.

Tool-assisted self manual therapy (TASMT)

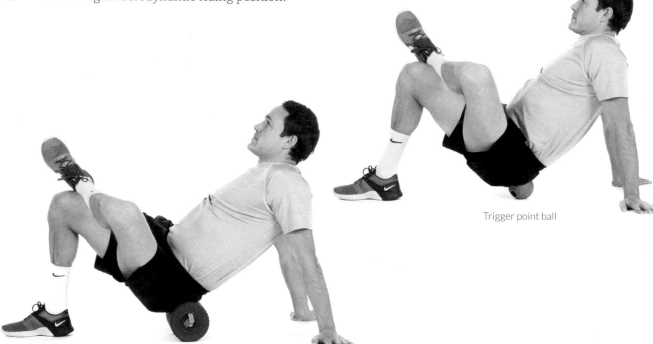

Trigger point ball

Foam roller

Anterior thigh opener

Returning to work on the quads, the muscles of the front of the thigh, this is a classic stretch that should be a mainstay for any cyclist. Although this is ostensibly a passive stretch, you'll get more benefit if you experiment with movement and shifting your bodyweight to discover areas of tightness. Once your body relaxes in one position, move slightly and, if necessary, try one of the more advanced options.

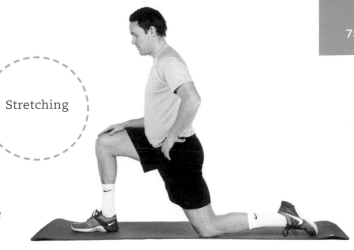

- From a kneeling position, bring your right leg forward so that you're in a kneeling lunge. You may find it more comfortable if your left knee is resting on a towel or mat.
- Make sure your right knee is directly over the right ankle and that your upper body is tall, with your centre of gravity over your kneeling left knee.
- Contract your trunk muscles without arching your back, squeeze your glutes and lean forward, increasing the flexion of your right leg and creating a stretch on your left hip and thigh.
- Allow the stretch to develop and intensify it by moving further forwards or by trying it with the rear leg elevated on a step or box.
- Repeat with the other leg.
- You can also try the banded option, placing the band after approximately 1 minute.

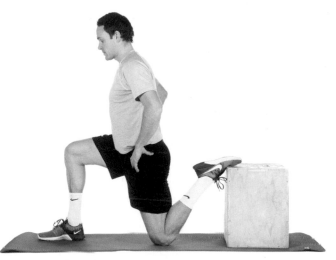

Rear foot elevated

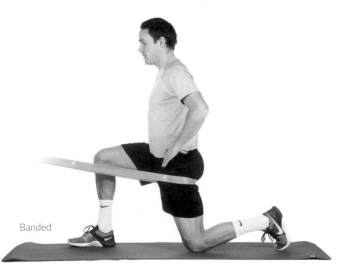

Banded

Posterior thigh opener

There is a huge variety of hamstring stretches but this is one of the most effective. Again, don't just hold a static stretch – this is an active exercise. Bend and straighten your leg to apply and release load.

Stretching

■ Lie on your back and loop a band around your left foot.

■ Bring your knee towards your chest.

■ Apply tension to your hamstring by straightening your knee. Increase the intensity by bending and straightening your leg.

■ Repeat with the other leg.

■ There is an option to apply an additional band to this stretch below.

Glute stretch

This is a great stretch for the glutes and a perfect one for doing in front of the TV.

Kneel on all fours and then bring your right leg through, placing it flat on the floor between your hands, with a 90-degree bend at the knee.

- Extend your left leg out behind you, rotating your knee under so that your knee and toes are on the floor.
- Sit back into the stretch, aiming for a straight and level pelvis. Your navel should be in line with the inside of your left thigh.
- Lift your chest up and breathe through the stretch.
- Experiment with dropping your chest down towards the floor and adding more rotation, gently working back and forth through any restrictions.
- Change sides and work on the other glute.
- If you struggle to get your hips straight, place a block under your hip
- You can also apply a band to this stretch.

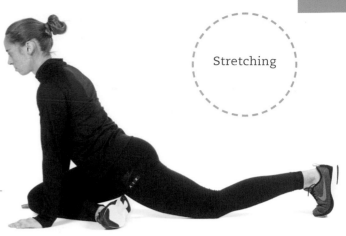

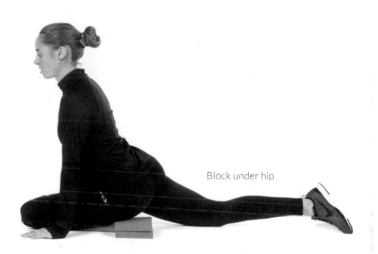

Block under hip

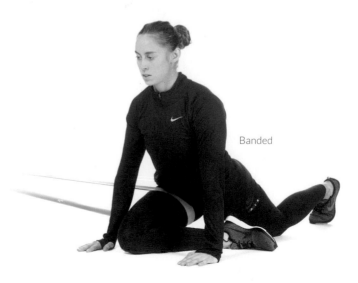

Banded

ROM: KNEE TO WALL CORRECTIVES

Tool-assisted self Manual therapy (TASMT)

Plantar fascia smash

The plantar fascia connects many of the complex and intricate muscles of the foot and ankle, and can easily become unyielding. This can lead to restriction in the surrounding muscles, pain and inflammation in the area, and have knock-on implications all the way up your lower body.

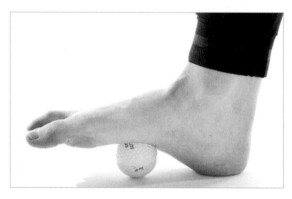

■ Standing in bare feet, use a golf ball or similar to roll around the sole of your foot. Apply as much pressure on to the ball as you feel you're able to.
■ Explore for tight or sore spots and, if you find one, oscillate on and off it for about 30–45 seconds or until you feel it release.
■ Move on to your other foot.
■ Some might find the pressure of performing this exercise standing too much. In this case, sit on a chair and reduce the amount of weight on the ball to a level you can handle.

Calf smash

Knee to wall can often be restricted by the muscles at the rear of the lower leg. Releasing both the gastrocnemius, the bulkier muscle at the top of your calves, and the soleus, the muscle that extends behind and below it, may help to restore normal range.

■ Adopt a seated position with a foam roller positioned mid-calf.
■ Support your bodyweight with your hands under your shoulders and elevate your buttocks off the ground.
■ Cross one ankle over the other to focus pressure on one calf.
■ Roll up and down the entire calf, explore for tight or sore spots and, if you find one, oscillate on and off it for about 30–45 seconds or until you feel it release.
■ Change sides and work on the other calf.
■ Circle and flex the ankle to get into different areas of the calf.
■ If a foam roller doesn't generate enough pressure, try a trigger point ball or similar.

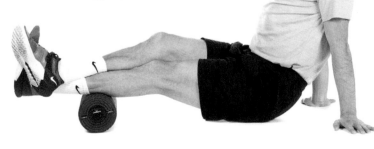

Ankle dorsiflexion opener

This exercise changes stretch tolerance in muscles surrounding the ankle joint, allowing movement into a fuller range.

■ Stand facing a wall with your hands flat against it at shoulder height to provide support and control. Your feet should be 30–45cm from the wall.

■ Step forward with your right foot, placing your heel as close to the bottom of the wall as possible and your toes and forefoot against the wall.

■ Rock up and forwards by coming up on your toes of the back (left) foot to develop a stretch in your right calf.

■ Move forwards and back, looking for particular areas of tightness in your calf and working through them.

■ Change sides to work on the left calf.

■ There are a number of options for band placement to facilitate this stretch.

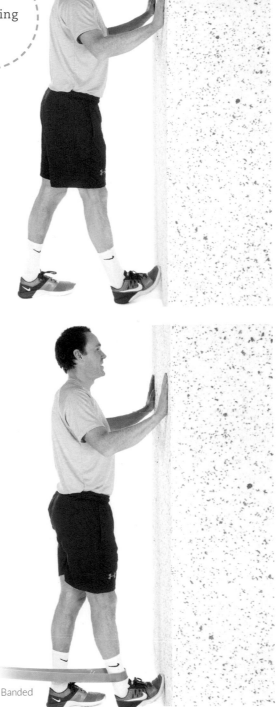

Banded

THORACIC SPINE

ROM: SITTING ROTATION CORRECTIVES

Thoracic spine extension smash

Extension and rotation are very closely linked in the thoracic spine – you can't have one without the other. That's why, with this exercise, we focus on creating more optimal thoracic extension as it's a great route to improved rotation. Extending over a foam roller, or a peanut if the large roller is too difficult, gives a good feeling of release after a long day on the bike or behind a desk.

■ Adopt a position as if you were about to perform sit-ups and position the foam roller or peanut under your back so that it's at the base of your ribcage.

■ Wrap your arms around yourself and actively pull your shoulders forward.
■ Extend over the roller by arching your back.
■ Spend time in this position until you feel change.
■ Come out of extension, keeping your arms wrapped around you, as if you're doing a sit-up. Allow your backside to move towards your feet, shifting the position of the roller further up your back.
■ Extend back over the roller and keep working in this way all the way up to the base of your neck.
■ Increase the extension and intensity by squeezing your glutes and pushing your hips up.

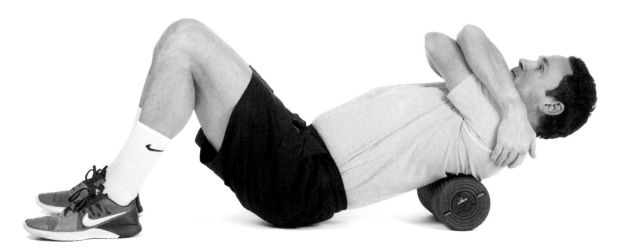

Side-to-side smash and roll

If you discover areas that aren't responsive to the straight extension exercise on the opposite page or you aren't seeing the improvements you want, try this side-to-side variant.

Tool-assisted self manual therapy (TASMT)

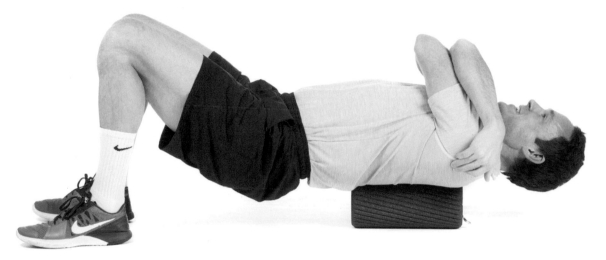

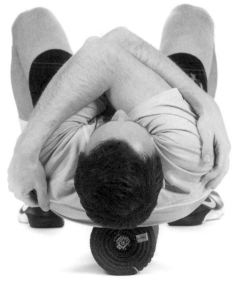

- Set up in the same way as the thoracic spine extension smash.
- Rather than extending over the foam roller, roll from side to side, keeping that tension on your upper back with your arms.
- Aim for as much rotation as possible.
- Work up your spine.
- If you find one side or area is especially tight, hold on it and roll up and down over it.
- Also try extending over the roller when on your side.
- This exercise is all about moving and exploring for tight or restricted areas. Don't be rigid and formulaic – be active and search them out.

Lats trigger ball release

This exercise could be used to improve all of the upper body assessments but we'll start with it here. The latissimus dorsi – 'lats' – has the largest single attachment of any muscle in the body. It's a key stabiliser not only of the shoulder but also, because of its extensive spinal insertions, of the spine. It often becomes restricted as, due to its size, the body recruits it to compensate for inactivity or weakness in other muscles. A lat of sufficient length and strength is key to many movements involving spinal rotation and overhead movement.

- Lying on a mat, extend one hand above your head.
- Insert a trigger point ball in your armpit near the insertion of your lat and rotator cuff.
- Roll over to put weight on the ball.
- Increase the amount of weight on the ball and move around the area to look for tight or restricted areas.
- You can also use a foam roller for this exercise.

> Tool-assisted self manual therapy (TASMT)

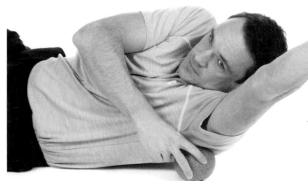

Placing the ball

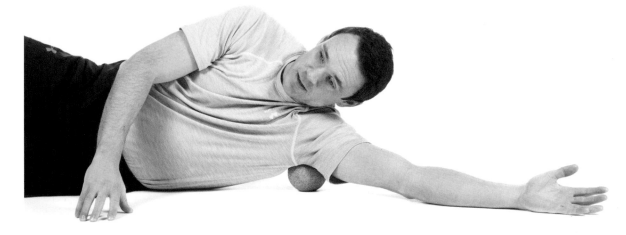

Recumbent kneeling lat stretch

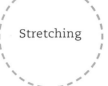

Stretching

As the lats are such large muscles, restrictions in them can have negative impacts both on and off the bike. Affecting both shoulder mobility and the spine, they are a key muscle group for good form in a huge number of common gym exercises, as well as achieving a good aerodynamic position on the bike.

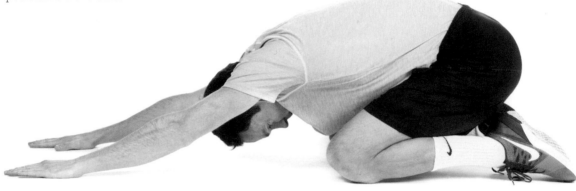

- Kneel and reach forward with your hands, placing them on the mat in front of you about shoulder-width apart.
- Keeping one hand where it is, place the other hand on top of it.
- Sit back gently towards your heels, making sure your hands stay in position.
- You should feel a stretch develop as you move backwards and, due to the hand position, should feel it on one side more than the other.
- Repeat with your hand position reversed.
- You can advance the stretch by side-bending away from the lower hand side or by elevating your hands on a bench or Swiss ball.

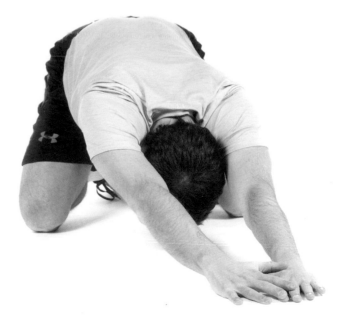

Seated spinal rotation

Thoracic rotation is a good indicator of thoracic extension. The latter is difficult to assess but, if rotation is good, in most cases extension will follow suit. Both thoracic rotation and extension are important in being able to achieve good movement patterns, as the thoracic region is effectively the link between the upper and lower body. Restrictions here can pass on unusual loads to other joints, both upwards and downwards, potentially resulting in overloading and breakdown. For example, a stiff thoracic spine often loads up the lumbar spine, resulting in lower back pain. A mobile and free-moving thoracic spine is a key component in realising a good riding position that doesn't place undue load elsewhere.

■ From a seated position with your legs extended forward, cross one foot across the opposite knee.
■ Bend the bottom leg to tuck your foot near the opposite hip.
■ Make sure your weight is evenly dispersed on both sides and, if necessary, use a towel or block to level them.
■ Sit tall and rotate towards your top leg. Aim to lock your elbow on the outside of the top leg.
■ Make sure you lead the stretch with your head and shoulders.

Stretching

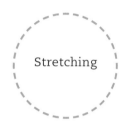

Shoulder rotator trigger point ball smash

The muscles at the front of the upper body often become tighter and more restricted, pulling us into an ever more stooped and rounded posture. We start life curled up in a ball and end up that way in our old age. They often become long, weak and restricted due to this and to the propensity of modern-day life to encourage us to spend significant time seated and hunched forwards. Getting into and releasing these structures can relieve shoulder pain, improve range of motion and enable better all-round posture. Performed regularly and well, this exercise will help you to achieve more internal and external rotation at the shoulder joint and therefore improve your performance in the Hands Behind Back test for which they are often the first limiting factor.

Tool-assisted self manual therapy (TASMT)

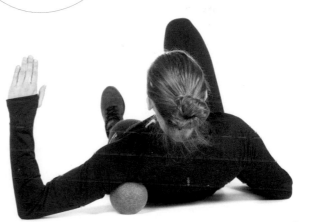

Positioning the ball

- Place a trigger point ball right above the insertion of your lat near your armpit.
- Lay back on to the ball with the arm on that side bent at 90 degrees. Put as much weight on to the ball as you feel comfortable with and adjust its position if necessary.
- Slowly rotate your arm forwards and back, aiming to increase the range of movement.

Trigger point ball pec release

Pec release work is a real double-edged sword. It's an amazingly rewarding exercise in terms of the payback and rewards in increased range of movement and decreased dysfunction, but it's normally incredibly painful. Simply lying on the trigger point ball is a great place to start and then, once you can cope with that, try the arm movements described below.

■ Lying on your front, position the trigger point ball so that it's nestled in the soft tissue between your shoulder and breastbone and below your collarbone.

■ Outstretch the arm on the side of the ball and hold the ball in place with the hand of your other arm.

■ Put as much weight as you can handle on to the ball.

■ If you feel you're able to, move your arm slowly above your head, by your side and behind your back.

■ Repeat on the other side.

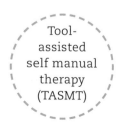

Tool-assisted self manual therapy (TASMT)

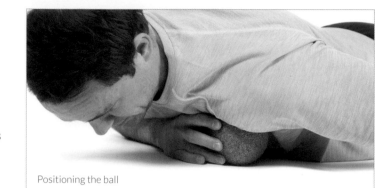

Positioning the ball

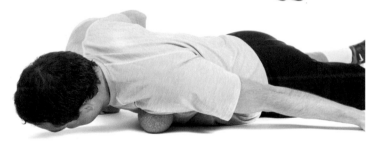

Start position

Arm movement

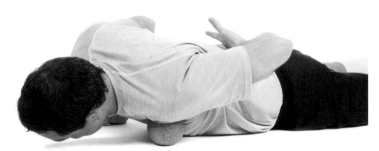

End position

Classic triceps/ lat stretch

Stretching

This stretch hits a number of structures including the long head of the triceps and the lats. Increasing your flexibility in this area will free up your shoulder in a way that's directly applicable to the Hands Behind Back assessment.

- Stand next to a wall and, with your left arm above your head, place your elbow and triceps against the wall.
- Lean into the wall and start to develop a stretch in your triceps.
- Grab the wrist of your left arm with your right hand and intensify the stretch by pushing your left hand towards your left shoulder.
- Repeat on the other side.
- You can further advance this exercise by introducing a trigger point ball and band distraction.

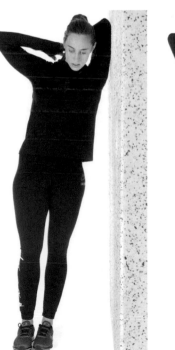
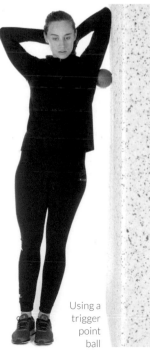

Using a trigger point ball

Reverse sleeper stretch

A fairly old-school stretch, but effective, and one you can do anytime and anywhere to work on internal shoulder rotation. If you're struggling with the hands behind back test, this is a stretch you can do at your desk regularly throughout the day and make real progress.

- In a seated, kneeling or standing position, put your left hand behind your back with your palm facing outwards.
- Reach across your body with your right hand and grab the elbow of your left arm.
- Without letting your right shoulder roll forwards or shrug up, pull your left elbow towards the centre line of your body.
- Repeat on the other side.

Stretching

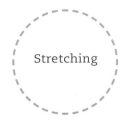

Aero gains 1

Even at this early stage of developing your range of movement you'll be working on a key factor that will directly improve your cycling performance, namely aerodynamics. It's only relatively recently that the importance of aerodynamics to cycling has become fully realised. Whereas once riders were looking for the lightest kit and components available, it's now known, in most riding scenarios, that aero trumps weight. Aero for cyclists is all about overcoming drag. Drag for a cyclist can be measured and expressed by a figure known as CdA. 'Cd' is the coefficient of drag. This is the resistance created by an object or shape when moving through the air. For example, a traditional round seat-tube will have a far higher coefficient of drag than an aero teardrop-shaped one. 'A' is the frontal area you present to the wind while moving forward on your bike. Aerodynamics are so important because the relationship between drag (expressed as CdA) and speed isn't linear. Simply put, doubling your power output doesn't double your speed or we'd see Tour de France sprinters battling for the line at over 250 kph. The reason this doesn't happen is that most of the energy you put into your pedals is used overcoming air resistance, hitting air molecules and punching them aside. As you go faster, not only are you hitting those air molecules harder but you're also having to push through more of them every second.

In the British Cycling 'Secret Squirrel Club', we were well ahead of the aero curve, spending hours testing in the wind tunnel, making mannequins of team riders and producing skinsuits so effective that the UCI banned them. However, for all the go-faster aero kit and equipment, the rider is accountable for 70–80 per cent of drag. If your position on the bike isn't aerodynamically optimised, you can't hold that position or it saps your power, you're wasting hard-earned watts and giving away speed.

Obviously, if you're targeting time trials or pursuit on the track, being able to get and hold aero is key, but it's also vital for road racers. Less obvious, maybe, is the importance for sportive riders. If you're able to hold an aero position and therefore expend less energy for the same speed on the flat, you'll have more left in the tank for climbs. Being able to get down and hold a position on your drops means faster and safer descending. Finally, in those last couple of hours of a gruelling ride, if you're not having to continuously sit up and stop pedalling to stretch your back out but can hold a strong aero position, you'll save significant time.

With all bike fits and positioning, the bike is infinitely adjustable and the rider is finitely adaptable. Often, because of the physical limitations of the rider, the bike has to be tweaked to accommodate these limitations, but this will always tend to involve compromising aerodynamic efficiency. Therefore, if you're able to adapt your body using the correctional exercises in this book, you'll be able to adopt a more aero position and hold it for longer. Over the last ten years we've managed to identify the key areas you should be working on and it's no coincidence that these are key areas of the assessment and subsequent exercises.

By focusing on these correctional exercises to improve your range of movement, you'll improve your ability to attain a more aerodynamic position on the bike. However, this isn't the end of the process and by working on your control and strength through that range of movement, you'll be able to sustain that position for longer, more stable in it and able to produce more power. We'll revisit aerodynamics in Chapter 4 and direct you towards your next set of exercises to enhance your aero gains.

1 **Pelvis** The most important area to look at regarding optimising aerodynamics is the pelvis. For most riders, getting aero means lowering their front end. If you can't rotate forwards at the pelvis, this has to be achieved from elsewhere in the body, often the lower back, known as the lumbar spine. This can lead to back pain, an inability to hold the position and, as the back is less flat from a lumbar bend, poorer aero-dynamics. Choice and orientation of saddle can be crucial in allowing your pelvis to rotate forwards but if your hamstrings and hip flexors are restricted, this will severely limit pelvis rotation and your ability to get low.

KEY EXERCISES
- Quad smash
- Hamstring smash
- Anterior thigh opener
- Posterior thigh opener

2 **Neck/cervical Spine** A function of dropping your front end is that your neck has to be able to extend more and more in order for you to be able to look down the road or track. Just try it – look straight up at the ceiling and try to hold this for a minute or more. The ability and strength to extend your neck is crucial for an optimal aero position and is largely dependent on your ability to extend your thoracic spine along with lat and pec flexibility.

KEY EXERCISES
- Thoracic spine extension smash
- Recumbent kneeling lat stretch
- Trigger point ball pec release

◀ *Improving your range of movement in key areas will improve your ability to attain a more aerodynamic position on the bike.*

3 **Upper back/thoracic spine** When discussing aerodynamic riding positions, the holy grail is a flatter back. Much of the ability to obtain a flatter back comes from the ability to rotate the pelvis but also crucial is how well you can extend through your thoracic spine.

KEY EXERCISES
- Side to side smash and roll
- Seated spinal rotation

4 **Shoulders** Along with getting low, the other factor for reducing frontal area and therefore drag is getting narrow. For this, good shoulder mobility is crucial.

KEY EXERCISES
- Shoulder rotator trigger point ball smash
- Banded shoulder distraction into extension and external rotation

Banded shoulder distraction into extension and external rotation

The shoulder is an amazing joint that, in combination with the elbow, wrist and fingers, allows for incredible dexterity in the arm. If you compare it with the body's other ball-and-socket joint, the hip, the difference in range of motions is fourfold. However, this motion comes at a cost, namely stability. It's very unusual to dislocate a hip but relatively common for shoulders. Even the act of trying to free up your shoulders can put them in potentially vulnerable positions. This is a great exercise as it allows you to work on two key ranges of motion, extension and external rotation, using your bodyweight but without any risk. It feels great after you've done it and encourages the shoulder joint towards the posterior part of the socket. This plays a significant role in correcting the 'shoulders rolled forwards' posture that is so common-place due to modern life.

- Attach a band to the wall/ceiling or similar at above head height.
- Hook your right hand through the band and then rotate your hand with palm up and thumb towards the outside of your body. This creates the external rotation.
- Place your right hand on top of your left hand and use it to hold the hand in the externally rotated position.
- Hinge and lower your torso towards the ground.
- Maintain the external rotation, contract and relax, and alter your body and foot position to search out and work through areas of restriction.
- Repeat on the other side.

Stretching

Find the exercises that work for you

The assessment will highlight the areas of your body that need work to develop range of movement and this chapter will point you in the direction of a number of exercise options to achieve that goal. As we're all individuals, we'll all respond differently to the various exercises and you'll need to experiment with the ones that feel best for you and have the greatest impact. Try different ones and varying combinations and keep referring back to the assessment to ascertain effectiveness.

Bite-sized chunks little and often

At this stage, the more regularly you can perform the exercises, the better. With daily work, or better still multiple times per day, you should make significant progress. You don't have to do a full routine every time – even 5–10 minutes performing a few exercises that you know work for you will be beneficial. On top of these daily doses, if you can also fit in two or three 20–30-minute dedicated sessions each week, that's the ideal. This sort of work shouldn't have any negative impact on your cycling workouts so can be scheduled in at any time.

Tool-assisted-self-manual-therapy (TASMT)

This uses a foam roller, trigger point ball or other tool to work on and release tight or restricted tissue. Typically, you'll use TASMT on an area to release it and then a stretching movement to develop range. It's important that you don't just mindlessly and passively roll back and forth over an area, but rather seek out and focus on tight and restricted areas.

Stretching

The exercises typically following TASMT have been designated as 'stretching' but this is only really for lack of another suitable term – 'degrees of freedom' or 'range developers' are a bit clunky! When following a stretching routine, you're not really making the muscle longer but are reducing a sensory response that's limiting its ability to move through its range.

Aero gains

If you have a competitive or impatient mindset, you might be finding it frustrating that your assessment results aren't allowing you to hit the gym and lift some heavy weights. However, aside from the fact that you're likely to be saving yourself some significant time on the physio's couch, you're already benefitting your cycling performance. Many of the exercises at this stage in the plan will enhance your ability to achieve a more aerodynamic position on your bike.

CONTROL THROUGH RANGE SUPPORTED CORRECTIVE EXERCISES

As we move on to control through range supported movements, we'll begin to introduce some exercises, alongside tool assisted self manual therapy and stretching, that will make your routine feel more like 'training'.

It's important at this stage that all of the exercises are performed in a precise manner and that you don't rush or cheat them in your enthusiasm to progress to loaded work. It's all too easy to develop bad habits at this stage, which will compromise your training as you move ahead. Take time to read through and understand the section below on lower back and pelvic control.

Remember, the assessment and its levels of corrective exercises isn't a one-way street with a final destination. It's a fluid process that will constantly move back and forth depending on your training, racing and variables outside of cycling. You should be constantly working through the assessment, using it and the exercises as a mobilisation routine and identifying the areas that need your focus and attention. Even if that means going back to Level 1 ROM corrective exercises, that's not a backwards step or a negative, it's just what your body requires at that moment.

THE IMPORTANCE OF LOWER BACK AND PELVIC CONTROL

The ability to control your trunk, especially the lumbar spine and pelvis, while executing movements is a fundamental building block for good, coordinated sustainable movement and loading. However, if you go into any gym or health club, you'll see people performing squats, dead lifts and overhead movements without this essential control and awareness. Rounding or excessive arching of the lower back are symptomatic of this issue, and to carry on loading in this flawed way is a recipe for long-term injury.

For this reason, lower back and pelvic control are key components to the assessment, especially during the active straight leg raise (ASLR) and overhead reach. However, whether consciously or not, it's possible to 'cheat' these movements. Being aware of this cheating, the reasons for it and how to eliminate it is vitally important as many people will, for example, be able to complete an ASLR but in a way that leaves them open to injury and limitation either through repeated exposure or when they load.

We don't believe in a perfect or normal way to move and many training and rehabilitation systems that try to pigeonhole people into these narrow prescriptive goals are ultimately destined to fail. The reason for this is that we're all individuals and we all move in slightly different ways. Ask 50 people to jump over a low wall and you'll observe a huge range of methods for completing this seemingly simple task. Ask them to jump off the wall and you'll see even more variety, as landing is actually a lot more demanding. The way people choose to jump the wall is governed by a huge number of factors. Previous experience of similar tasks,

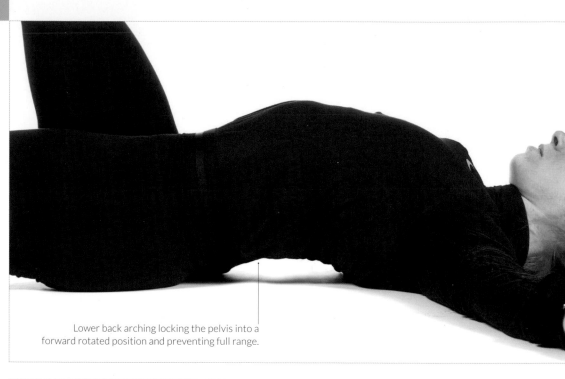

Lower back arching locking the pelvis into a
forward rotated position and preventing full range.

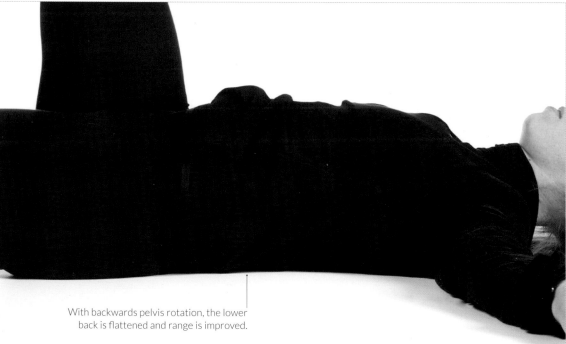

With backwards pelvis rotation, the lower
back is flattened and range is improved.

different degrees of freedom and varying control and strength across joints are just some of them. We don't have to consciously think about it, our bodies find the best way for us to complete it.

It's the same when we're recovering from an injury. A classic example is a twisted ankle. When we're healthy we'll probably bound down a flight of steps, but with a damaged ankle we'd take one step at a time, maximising the use of our good foot. This modification to our movement pattern facilitates rest and healing but allows us to continue living our day-to-day life. As the injury heals, our body adjusts and we gradually return to a more normal movement pattern.

However, this incredible ability of our bodies to adapt and compromise to perform movements can lead to problems and the 'cheating' we've alluded to. Some areas of the body are more susceptible to a creeping and gradual loss of freedom of movement and strength and control. These areas are often the more complex, multi-small-joint units, such as the lumbar spine and pelvis. Their complex multi-joint nature gives them a huge amount of scope for adaptation and compensation. If the ideal combination of joints isn't able to perform a movement optimally, others will take up the slack and find a way around the problem. This isn't necessarily a problem in isolation or infrequently, but if this cheat or short cut is constantly relied upon, it will be hardwired and become the norm.

Taking this back to the ASLR, a common limiting factor in achieving full range is an inability of the pelvis to posteriorly rotate, which prevents the hip and leg flexing and extending properly. Unless you have a

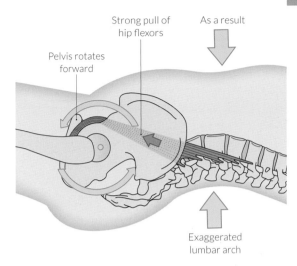

Strong pull of hip flexors

As a result

Pelvis rotates forward

Exaggerated lumbar arch

▲ How tight hip flexors can rotate the pelvis into a forward rotated position, cause a lumbar arch and limit range.

background in physiotherapy, this language and concept can be quite hard to grasp so it's best explained in pictures.

As you can see, the athlete in the first photo is struggling to reach 75 degrees of elevation with their ASLR. If we zoom in, you can see why. Their lower back (lumbar region) is arched off the floor, effectively locking the pelvis into an anterior or forward rotated position and preventing full range.

In the second photo, the athlete has managed to rotate their pelvis posteriorly or backwards, which has the effect of flattening their back against the floor and allows an improvement in their ASLR range.

You can easily demonstrate this on yourself. Perform an ASLR as described in Chapter 2 and note when you feel a pull on the back of your knee and hamstrings. Now do the same again but place one or two small cushions in the small of your back to create an arch. You'll find that you probably feel the pull earlier and are able to achieve less range.

A lot of people lose the ability to posteriorly rotate their pelvis. A sedentary lifestyle, even time spent on the bike, can contribute to this but the causes are numerous. It could be pain or stiffness in the lumbar spine inhibiting the movement into a flat position. There could be a lack of strength or control to attain and then hold the position, or a lack of range or tightness in another joint – the hip flexors, for example – could be pulling the lumbar spine into an arch.

However, because of our body's ability to adapt, compensate and cheat, some people are able to achieve a passable ASLR without posterior pelvic rotation. A common cheat is using inhaled air to depress the diaphragm and effectively brace the lumbar spine against the floor. The pelvis hasn't rotated backwards, it has followed the spine there. Fortunately, we have ways to expose such cheats and, in the case of the ASLR, it's the raise and lower. By loading the movement, just with the weight of the leg, those lacking the strength and control to hold the pelvis rotated backwards and the lumbar spine flat against the floor will see the back arch into extension as the leg lowers.

You will discover any such issues during the assessment process, be able to correct them and develop an understanding and awareness of your lumbar-pelvis positioning. You will then be able to move on to more advanced loaded movements, such as squats, confident that you're not loading a narrow-based pyramid of limited range, poor control and low strength, leading to pain and potential back injuries. Your form and movement doesn't have to be perfect but some ways to achieve movements and tasks are definitely better than others – just take a look round the gym next time you go.

HIP, LUMBAR SPINE, PELVIS AND LEG

CONTROL THROUGH RANGE SUPPORTED: ACTIVE STRAIGHT LEG RAISE AND LOWER CORRECTIVES

The exercises prescribed for the active straight leg raise (ASLR) correctives in Chapter 2 are still appropriate if you're unable to successfully complete the active straight leg raise and lower. However, for the lowering component of the exercise, and to develop the necessary pelvic control and awareness to allow you to successfully complete it, you should additionally focus on the exercises below.

Pelvic positioning awareness developer

As we've just discussed, developing good pelvic positioning awareness and control is essential for progression through this plan and that's why it's prioritised at this early stage. Getting this exercise right and under control lays the foundations for the strong stable base that we then start to load later in the plan.

■ Lie on your back and place one or both of your hands underneath your lumbar spine.
■ Rotate your pelvis backwards to flatten your back against your hands, squashing them slightly. This can be hard to initiate or envisage, so think about these cues. Imagine trying to curl your groin round towards your navel without lifting your buttocks off the floor. Alternatively, think about squeezing your buttocks to push them along the floor away from you. When you get these cues right, you will feel gentle pressure develop on your hands from your lower back.
■ First practise generating the pressure and then progress to holding it.
■ Avoid holding your breath, as this fills the diaphragm with air and creates a false feeling of pressure. This common 'cheat' is a compromised solution to developing control and breaks down as soon as you breathe out, something that's unavoidable.
■ To prevent breath-holding, count aloud or go through the alphabet. If you're doing it right, there should be no change in the pressure on your hands.
■ Once you're confident with the action and are able to maintain pressure on your hands, progress the exercise.
■ Set up a posterior pelvic tilt by following the steps previously described and, once stable, straighten one leg away from you, keeping the heel on the floor.
■ As you extend the leg, you will feel your lumber spine wanting to extend away from the floor and the pressure on your hands reduce.
■ Counter this by maintaining the posterior pelvic tilt, utilising the cues described above.
■ Perform 5–10 slow and controlled reps with one leg and then repeat with the other.

Single leg supported leg lowers

Once you have used the previous exercise to develop your awareness of pelvic positioning, the next stage is to learn to control your pelvis while under load.

■ Lie on your back in a doorway with one leg next to the frame and, having moved your backside towards the door frame, straighten and rest your other leg against the frame in a position where you feel a light stretch on your hamstrings.

■ The leg not on the door frame will still be straight on the floor.

■ Ensure you have both hands out at your side with your palms up or, if you need feedback to maintain a neutral spine, have your hands slightly under your lower back and maintain pressure on them.

■ Focusing on keeping your lower back in contact with the floor, perform a straight leg raise with the leg not against the door.

■ Pause at the top of the movement, forcefully exhale through the mouth as if inflating a balloon and lower the leg to the floor with no change in spinal position.

■ Repeat until your form fails or you manage 10 reps (see instructions below) and then change to the other leg.

■ If you're unable to perform 1 rep, use a step, a stack of cushions or similar to reduce the range of the exercise so you aren't lowering completely to the floor.

■ Aim to build up to a set of 10 reps and perform 3–5 sets.

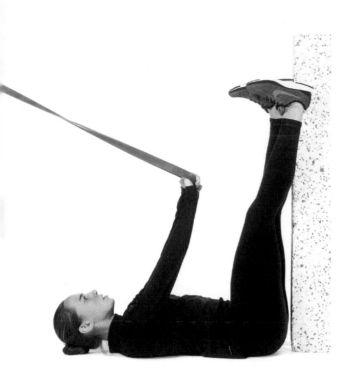

Single leg lowering with core engagement

Once awareness of pelvic positioning and control has been developed using the previous exercises, the next step is to be able to control the pelvis under load. This progression increases the load from the single leg supported leg lowers by reducing the amount of support. The band helps to facilitate a greater contraction of the abdominal muscles.

■ Lie on your back with your head next to a wall or frame that allows you to attach a band for the pulldowns.
■ Focusing on pelvic positioning and keeping your lower back in contact with the floor, perform a straight arm pulldown, bringing your arms down by your sides.
■ Maintaining your arm position and lower back contact, elevate both legs.
■ Working on one leg, lower and raise it. Don't take it all the way to the ground – aim for a few centimetres off.
■ Aim for 10 reps and then change to other leg and repeat.
■ Once you're able to manage 10 reps on each side, you should be able to perform the active straight leg raise and lower required in the assessment.

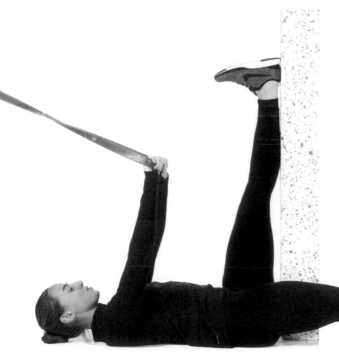

THORACIC SPINE

CONTROL THROUGH RANGE SUPPORTED: WALL OVERHEAD REACH CORRECTIVES

If you have achieved a pass in both the hands behind back and sitting rotation tests, there shouldn't be too much more to address. However, if you're still lacking some range of movement, there's little point in starting to work on control. So, we start off with a few additional range developing exercises that will help you achieve the overhead reach.

Tool-assisted self manual therapy (TASMT)

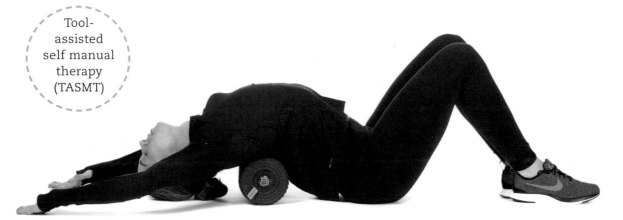

Thoracic extension and overhead reach with foam roller

Similar to earlier exercises for thoracic spine extension and rotation, this can easily be included in the same sequence. It has the additional mobilising effect of extending your arms overhead at the same time as extending your thoracic spine.

■ Lie in a sit-up position with the base of your ribcage on a foam roller.

■ Raise your arms overhead and extend over the foam roller. The extension should come from your thoracic spine; take care to maintain a neutral lumbar spine.

■ Take your arm to fully overhead and increase pressure by raising your hips.

■ Start lower down the thoracic spine and work up, discovering and focusing on where you feel most restricted in getting your arm above your head.

■ Retry the overhead reach test after doing this exercise – you may be pleasantly surprised.

First rib mobilisation

The first rib is an almost magical point in the body for physical therapists. In releasing it, either through passive treatment or active mobilisation, we always see impressive returns. It not only has a key mechanical role as the juncture between the cervical and thoracic spine but also has a bearing on the shoulder. Directly beneath it lies a veritable trunk road of nerves, the brachial plexus, which contains the vast majority of nerves serving the upper limbs and body. This explains why it can be so important in overall shoulder and thoracic spine mobility as, if this area is tight or restricted, all the neural elements will be anchored and bound down. Freeing up this structure can be a genuine awakening moment for many people.

■ Locate the soft recess between your collar-bone and the base of your neck. This is where you'll be placing the trigger point ball.

■ With a looped band and holding the ball under the band, sling the band over your right shoulder.

■ Hold the ball and band in place and bend down to hook the other end of the band over your left foot.

■ Stand up slowly, creating tension on the band and pressure on the ball.

■ Raise and rotate your right arm, perform arm circles and look away with your head. Explore movement, looking for areas of restriction and working through them.

■ Change to work the other side.

Tool-assisted self manual therapy (TASMT)

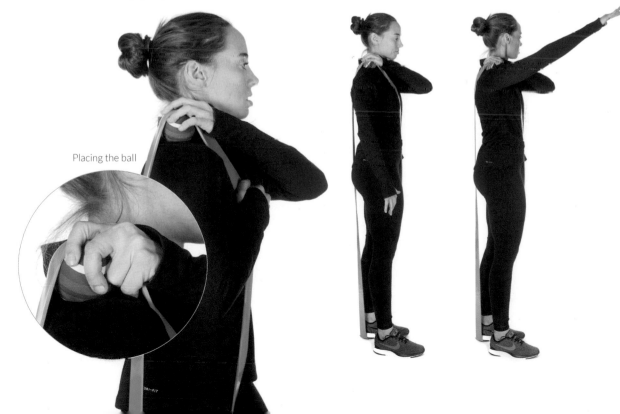

Placing the ball

Glute smash with foam roller

Tool-assisted self manual therapy (TASMT)

One of the stop points for the overhead reach test is not maintaining contact with the wall with your lower back. Although you may achieve the required range with your arms, not being able to control your lumbar spine and arching is significant. It indicates that your ability to posteriorly rotate your pelvis may be the limiting factor.

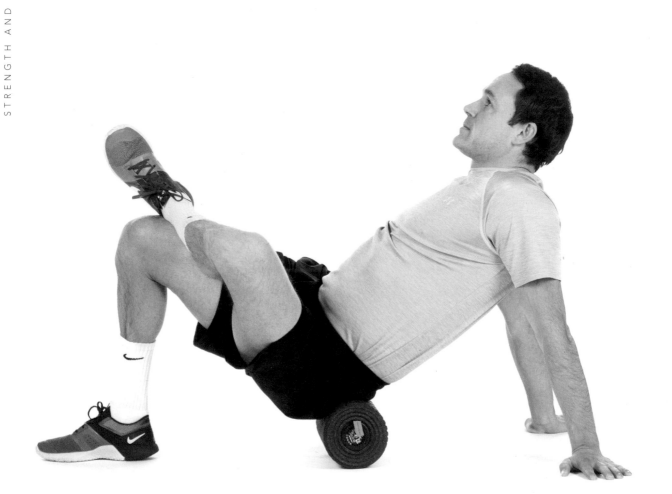

Hump and hollow stretch

The four-point kneeling hump and hollow exercise, also known as the cat and cow, is an old standard but it's nonetheless tried, tested and effective. It's great for helping you feel and understand what it is to anteriorly and posteriorly tilt your pelvis while performing other movements. The final moment of the exercise is exactly the same as trying to hold your pelvis back and lumber spine against the wall while reaching overhead. However, the kneeling position provides more support so you can focus on the elements most likely to be limiting.

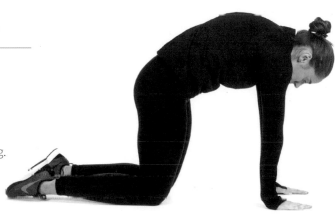

- Adopt a four-point kneeling position with your knees under your hips and your hands under your shoulders.
- Create a hump by rounding your back. Imagine there's a rope going through your navel and it's being pulled towards the ceiling.
- Create the hollow by imagining that the rope is now being pulled towards the floor, arching your back and driving your buttocks high.
- Slowly alternate between the two positions three or four times, allowing the stretch to develop in each position.
- The movement should come just from your lumbar spine and pelvis; there should be no bending of your arms or shifting your legs away from the hips-above-knees alignment.
- Finish the exercise by holding the hump position and then slowly sitting back on your heels while maintaining the posteriorly tilted pelvis.

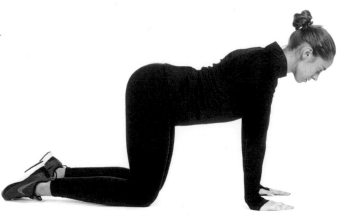

Pilates and yoga

Pilates is named after its founder, Joseph Pilates, who developed it as a rehabilitation system for injured dancers. Genuine Pilates uses a reformer machine, a sliding bench with springs for resistance. It allows the development of range to attain the positions involved in the exercises and then the strength to control and hold them against the resistance. The term 'yoga' covers a huge range of styles including hot Bikram, gentle Hatha and energetic Ashtanga. Both Pilates and yoga will certainly develop and challenge your movement range and add to your broad base of conditioning. An additional benefit of both is the focus on breathing, which, as cyclists, you can only benefit from working on.

If you're considering trying Pilates or yoga, the key is to find the right class and instructor. There's a massive difference between a small Pilates reformer class with a qualified instructor and a 30-person mat class overseen by someone who's only done a weekend course. The exercises and poses in both Pilates and yoga are very precise and the smallest adjustment can make all the difference. A number of riders on the Great Britain Cycling Team include Pilates and yoga in their training but we'll do everything we can to ensure the quality of the class, instructor and their technique. You should do the same, and our advice, especially if you're a novice, would be to invest in some one-to-one instruction before moving on to bigger group classes.

Both Pilates and yoga can be excellent complementary activities to cycling and the exercises in this book. Certainly, if you're more likely to attend a class rather than working out at home in a cold garage or spare room, it's a no-brainer and can be a great way to motivate yourself to a focused session of off the bike work. Use the assessment to determine your weaknesses and to see how the Pilates or yoga you're doing is helping you to progress. You'll probably notice we've drawn on them both when prescribing our exercises. This cross-pollination of ideas and an openness to other ways of thinking is essential for developing holistic, balanced and effective training and treatment plans. Nothing is truly original and if you find a trainer, practitioner or guru who claims their way is the only way, be wary.

◀ *Both Pilates and yoga can be excellent complementary activities to cycling and the exercises in this book.*

Control through range

Having spent time developing your range of movement, it's vital to be able to control your limbs and body through that range. Some people are born with extremely mobile joints but lack strength and control. They may display full range of movement and have the degrees of freedom for squatting, but if you placed a loaded barbell on their shoulders, it could be disastrous. Similarly, if you've had to spend time developing your range, you'll now have to add control.

Lower back and pelvic control

Our bodies are brilliant at finding ways to allow us to move and perform actions even if we lack the capability to do them optimally. This is great from a survival perspective but not always so good for conditioning and long-term health. If you load a compromised or 'cheat' movement, you're compounding it and, rather than widening your base of conditioning, are effectively narrowing it. Lower back and pelvic control is a common area where many people develop cheat mechanisms that can impact significantly on a range of movements and exercises. Fortunately, the assessment and exercises will allow you to identify and correct these cheats.

Pilates and yoga

It's no coincidence that you'd perform some of the exercises in this book in both Pilates and yoga classes, and both of these activities can be excellent for cyclists and can be very complementary to this plan. If you're thinking of starting either of them, do some research, find a recommended and qualified instructor, and invest in some one-to-one sessions to get you started.

CONTROL THROUGH RANGE UNSUPPORTED CORRECTIVE EXERCISES

As you move on to this level, the exercises will feel even more like training than during the control through range supported phase. We'll start talking more about sets and reps and, especially once we start introducing load, you'll need to start thinking more about how these sessions are scheduled in.

If you're fairly new to strength training, you'll find that almost any stimulation of your muscles will lead to progress. For this reason, it's not necessary to focus too much on the amount of weight or the number of reps and sets you're achieving. As you progress, these factors will become more important but for now the priority should be developing good technique. It's also important to remember that it's not just your muscles that are being strengthened. Tendons and ligaments, collectively referred to as connective tissues, will also be slowly adapting to your new training routine. Connective tissue adaptation tends to lag behind muscles and, although you might feel as though you're stronger and capable of lifting more, upping the load too quickly could put these tissues at risk of injury.

Rather than the daily bite-sized and even multiple times per day work that you might have been doing for the tool-assisted self manual therapy (TASMT) and stretching exercises of the earlier levels, you should now be looking at two or three dedicated sessions per week if you're in a phase of your training where you're focusing on off the bike conditioning. Try to adhere to the following guidelines:

■ Perform the exercises at least twice a week, with 48 hours between sessions. You can still work on your TASMT and stretching exercises on top of these sessions.
■ Choose the exercises that are specific to you, as determined by the assessment.
■ Ensure that you are performing the exercise correctly. Developing good form and technique should take priority over load.
■ Use the RPE scale to select load. See below for full guidelines.

You will also need to consider how these sessions may impact on your on the bike workouts and vice versa. Trying to combine endurance training and strength-focused training is known as concurrent training and can be problematic to manage. Training to improve endurance outcomes at the same time as trying to improve resistance exercises can be detrimental to the overall outcome. This is an area of considerable research and controversy but it basically boils down to placing the cells of the body under conflicting demands. Typically, endurance exercise affects the outcome of resistance training more so than RT does endurance exercise. There are many contributing factors to consider, such as the frequency and mode of endurance exercise and its duration. Of all endurance activities, cycling typically causes the lowest interference with strength gains due to its very low impact levels and consequently very low levels of muscle damage. However, if you're trying to combine high-intensity cycling workouts and heavy resistance training for a period of time, they can have a negative impact on one another. There are a number of steps you can take to minimise the interference effect.

■ Maximise recovery time between endurance and resistance training. If possible, schedule your training to allow at least 8 hours. So, for example, a split day with a cycling workout at 0800 in the morning and then a resistance session at 1800 would be fine.

▼ *Endurance and resistance training can impact negatively on each other so you need to consider both recovery and training structure.*

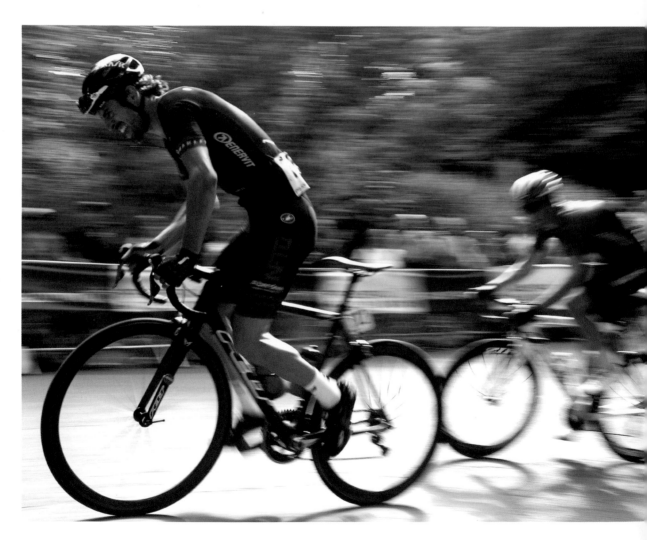

■ Optimise refuelling between sessions. Make sure to use a recovery drink or have a meal containing both protein and carbohydrates after training sessions and in the lead-up to the second session.

■ Strength first. While far from ideal, if you're unable to separate resistance and endurance work into separate sessions, do the resistance training first.

■ Don't lift to failure. When resistance training, avoid training to failure. Pushing to this point greatly increases the amount of recovery time needed and any potential strength gains are not offset by this.

In reality, if you're focusing on resistance training, your cycling performance in the short term is likely to suffer. This is why the off season is the best time to concentrate on your off the bike conditioning. Also, as the volume and intensity of your cycling is likely to be lower, you should experience better gains from your resistance training.

RPE SCALE

Part of this progression to a more 'training' feel to the exercises, as opposed to a corrective one, is an understanding of rated perceived exertion (RPE). As a cyclist, it's likely that you may be familiar with the concept of RPE and have used it to gauge effort during your cycling. You will probably have referred to the 20-point Borg scale, which, in conjunction with both heart rate and power, provides a powerful tool for cardiovascular exercise. However, RPE can also be a useful tool for strength training. Rather than having to perform a one-rep max for an exercise, which is fraught with difficulty

and potentially danger, and calculate loads for rep ranges based on that, once you are familiar with using RPE, it provides a safe but effective alternative. It's also very well suited to body-weight movements such as press-ups and inverted rows.

RPE SCORE	SENSATION
< 5.5	Too easy to count as a true work set
6	Fairly easy, would be good as a warm-up set
6.5	Borderline warm-up set
7	Lifting/movement speed fairly quick, would be good as an easy opening set
7.5	Could have MAYBE done 3 more reps
8	Could have DEFINITELY done 2 more reps
8.5	Could have MAYBE done 2 more reps
9	Could have DEFINITELY done 1 more rep
9.5	Could have MAYBE done 1 more rep
10	DEFINITELY unable to do another rep

Where appropriate in this and the following chapter, we will make recommendations regarding the RPE you should be looking to achieve for given exercises. RPE is good because, rather than working towards a blind rep target, it encourages body awareness. Remember, completing a set is not just about getting through the reps however you can – if your form breaks down, that should be the end of that set.

HIP, LUMBAR SPINE, PELVIS AND LEG

CONTROL THROUGH RANGE UNSUPPORTED: HIP HINGE CORRECTIVES

For the hinge, or any complex multi-joint exercise, the key to good technique is learning and hardwiring how to perform the movement correctly. This involves rehearsing and practising it with various cues. As you probably won't have a coach to give you pointers, external cues with biofeedback are probably the best teach-yourself options.

External cues are ones that direct the athlete's attention away from their body and towards the effects of their movements on their environment. Biofeedback refers to things that provide sensory information that allows an athlete to complete the movement well. In this context, this could be a stick down the back, using a wall or another method. The key is that they're tangible and easy-to-understand cues for the athlete, rather than vague notions of how a movement should feel. In our experience, external cueing tends to work better with cyclists and other athletes as it gives them multiple chances to experience and practise the movement. With any movement that is not routinely performed, a lack of body awareness will tend to be the main limiting factor.

For any hinging activity, the key points to be aware of are:

Keep your back flat/ neutral and maintain good pelvic positioning

Create horizontal separation from your hips and shoulders

Pull your chest forwards

Push your hips back

Don't let your knees track forwards, press them back

Similar to the corrective exercises at earlier levels, there is a need for some trial and error to find the drill that you best connect with. Remember, we're all individuals and we all respond to different cueing strategies. Don't forget the option of videoing yourself or getting a training partner to do so. By reviewing yourself, this will generally increase the effectiveness of any strategy.

Once you have found the exercise or exercises that work best for you from the first three (under the heading 'Developing the pattern'), regular repetition is the key to progression. Aim to perform 3 sets of 10 reps daily until you can consistently perform the hinge as per the assessment guidelines. Once you can achieve this, you should move on to the last two exercises to cement the pattern. At this stage, follow the set/rep guidelines for the exercise and the scheduling guidelines earlier in the chapter.

Hands down thigh hinge

For some people, sliding the hands down the thighs while maintaining the posture outlined in the key hinging points above can be a quick and simple way to learn the hinge pattern.

Developing the pattern

- Stand tall with soft knees and vertical shins.
- Slide your hands down your thighs, without allowing the knees to travel forward.
- With each rep, try to push the hips back slightly further without losing your flat back or letting the knees creep forward.

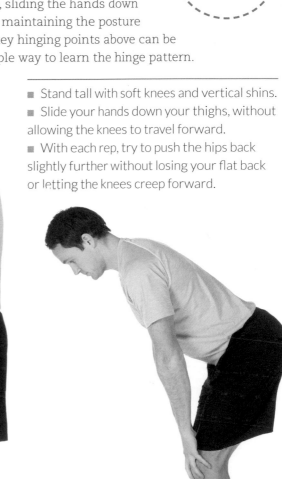

Stick down the back hinge

In effect a rehearsal or practice of the hinge assessment, the stick is useful if you have poor awareness of spinal position as it gives you feedback on where your back is.

■ Stand upright with your feet approximately shoulder-width apart and with straight but not locked knees.

■ Hold a dowel as shown in the image above. The key contact points that must be maintained throughout the exercise are: Dowel touching back of head, upper hand touching back of neck, dowel touching upper back, lower hand touching lower back and dowel touching tailbone.

■ Hinge by pushing your hips backwards. Your knees can bend slightly.

■ With each rep, assuming you're maintaining full contact with the stick, aim for slightly more depth until you're consistently hitting the 50-degree torso bend demanded by the assessment.

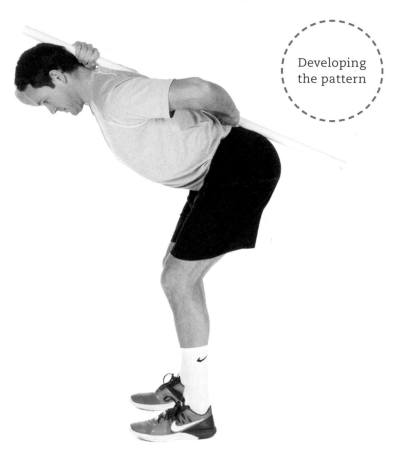

Developing
the pattern

Bum to wall hinge

This exercise is particularly useful if you struggle with creating horizontal separation from hips to shoulders as it gives you a tangible target and ensures that the movement comes from the hips.

■ Stand with your back to a wall and with your heels touching the wall, then step one foot distance away from the wall.

■ Keeping soft knees, hinge, keeping a flat back, until your backside touches the wall.

■ Pause in the touch position to feel the stretch on your hamstrings and to perform a scan of the key coaching points for the hinge.

Developing the pattern

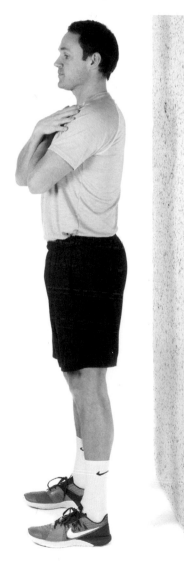

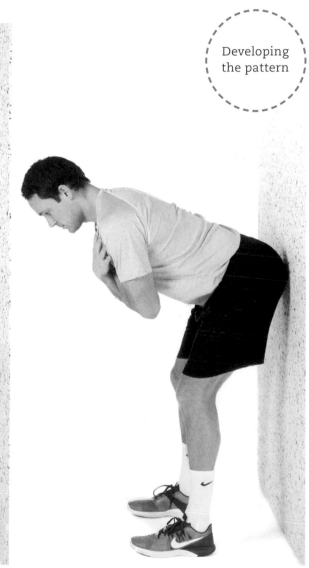

CONTROL THROUGH RANGE UNSUPPORTED CORRECTIVE EXERCISES

Static hold loaded hinge

Once you can consistently perform the hinge pattern without load, it is necessary to cement or hardwire the pattern into your neurological framework. If you don't complete the next two steps and keep them as part of your regular training, your ability to hinge will diminish quickly. External loading is useful for this as it gives your body a reason to remember the movement pattern and it also starts to strengthen the muscles, bones and connective tissue through the body.

Adding external load to the hinge can be achieved using a kettlebell, dumbbell, weighted rucksack or a plate. The key in this exercise is that the load is kept over the upper abs and sternum as this raises the centre of mass and helps the attainment of the desired position.

Cementing the pattern

- Holding an appropriate load, perform a hinge.
- Brace and hold at the bottom of the movement, ensuring you maintain all the key hinge coaching points.
- Hold the position for the times indicated below, return to the start position, pause and repeat for the given number of repetitions.

3 sets of 5 x 5 seconds, adjusting load to make it challenging (7–8 RPE).

Loaded hinge

Cementing
the pattern

Once you can consistently achieve the static hold loaded hinge, you are then ready to progress to the next level of external loading, which is to start to move more dynamically. This will continue to cement the movement pattern and start to prepare your body for the hinging movements associated with more complex movements such as squats.

■ Holding an appropriate load in the same way as for the static hold loaded hinge, hinge up and down following the guidelines below.
■ Once confident in your ability to hinge with the centrally held load, progress to holding the load in your hands using kettlebells, dumbbells or a barbell. This will require greater control of the movement.

Progression 1
3 x 5 reps with a 4-second lower, 2-second pause at the bottom of the movement and controlled lift (7–8 RPE).

Progression 2
3 x 10 reps with a normal smooth land-controlled lifting tempo (7–8 RPE).

You should perform Progression 1 until you are comfortable and confident with the pattern under load as, by slowing the movement down, it allows for more control. Moving to Progression 2 increases the velocity of the movement.

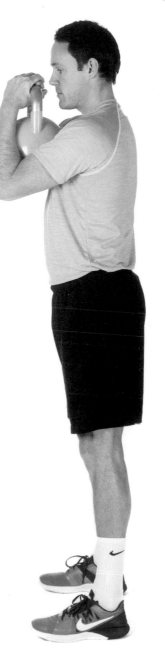

CONTROL THROUGH RANGE UNSUPPORTED: SQUAT CORRECTIVES

The squat is the classic exercise for many people when talking about enhancing cycling performance. It can be a great exercise when done correctly but you need to earn the right to perform it and load it. Too many generic off the bike training plans prescribe loaded squatting with little or no consideration given to whether the athlete has sufficient movement capabilities. Only once you have sufficient range and control of the various joints involved should you think about using it as part of a performance plan.

The squat can be loaded in a number of different ways, which changes the exercise slightly, but at its heart there are more similarities than differences. For example, a front squat (where the bar is placed across the front of the shoulders) increases the amount of contribution from the quadriceps in comparison with a more commonly performed back squat. However, there are a number of key/common elements required for successful performance of the lift.

To the right are the key points of squatting, working from the ground up. It's important to note that squatting is a full body activity and that it is the summation of all these points that will lead to successful performance of the squat.

Foot position is critical as it is the point of contact with the floor, which ultimately is where force must be applied. The feet should be set up in a stance that allows you to feel strong and stable; for the majority of people, this is around shoulder-width apart. When squatting, the feet should be flat on the floor. They can be turned out – recommendations vary widely on this and there are arguments

Head should be looking forwards. Avoid excessive arching

The knees should stay aligned to the feet

Exact width, 'flaring' and position of the feet is very much down to the individual. However, the key is feeling strong and stable and then 'screwing' your feet into the floor

Depth should be appropriate to your ability

for more 'flare' and less 'flare' (i.e. how turned out the feet are). In our experience, the width of the stance and the foot flare should be determined by the individual and should allow them to feel strong and stable or connected to the floor. It is commonly thought that the stance should be symmetrical; however, given the vast differences in human anatomy (even within the same person), it is our opinion that the stance need not be symmetrical and again should be dictated by the individual (as per above).

Once a comfortable position has been found, the feet should be 'screwed into the floor'. A simple cue is to imagine you are standing on a piece of paper on the floor. Once you have found your stance, you try to tear the paper with your feet. This activates the lower limb and trunk musculature and prepares it for the activity to come.

Maintaining the proper position of the spine, including the head, during squatting is critical. Again, there is much discussion around what is the optimal spinal position. Traditional lifting 'textbooks' taught a hard lumbar arch; however, when this is loaded it can be problematic for some athletes as it places load on structures that are not designed to be loaded (i.e. loads into an extended position). Everyone has a unique body position/size/shape and therefore their optimal position will also be unique. The best way is to create three-dimensional stability, which involves the interaction of the whole body rather than focusing on a specific area. An analogy to explain this is through the guy ropes on a tent – each one providing the 'optimal' amount of tension to create a balanced structure.

The goal when squatting (descending) is to maintain this position while flexing the hips and knees. When descending and ascending, the knees should stay aligned with the feet – otherwise you end up loading structures that are not designed to be loaded. An example of a common fault is valgus collapse, where the knees cave in towards each other. This ends up loading the knee joint in an inappropriate manner, which can cause inflammation and pain.

Depth of the squat should then be dictated by the ability to maintain the appropriate body positions. If you can't maintain optimal alignment at the foot, knee, hip and spine, what's the point in squatting deeper? At the end of the day, you are trying to use the squat to enhance performance by loading the various muscles and joints involved in a way that will provide a strengthening stimulus. If you don't follow these technique guidelines or load in a way that prevents you from doing so, you are exceeding the capabilities of your body, which can lead to trauma/damage, inflammation and possibly even injury. This then has the opposite effect to what you are trying to achieve (i.e. improve health and performance).

In the same way as with the hinge, we will be using the first three exercises to develop the squat pattern and then, by progressing to the last two exercises, where load is introduced, cementing the pattern.

Bodyweight squat with arms in front

Developing the pattern

By removing the dowel across the shoulders that we used for the squat in the assessment, it allows you to use your arms as a counter-balance and gives you the opportunity to get a real feel for the movement.

■ Adopt a standing position and, following the key squatting guidelines on pages 116-117, find a strong and stable position at the foot, ankle, hip and shoulder. Use this exercise as an opportunity to experiment with your squat starting position and to determine the foot width and alignment that feels best for you.

■ Not forgetting to screw your feet into the floor, once you've found your solid position, slowly descend into a squat with your arms out in front of you. Go as deep as you feel you're able to while maintaining good form.

■ Pause at the bottom and, without locking your knees, return to the start position and repeat.

■ Although you can try to sense your form, or observe it in a mirror, if possible have someone observe or video your squat. You can then look for the points where you divert from the optimal alignments at the foot, knee or trunk.

3 x 5 reps of slow lower (4 seconds) with isometric pause (2 seconds) at the bottom of the movement.

The pause will increase awareness of your body in space and help to reinforce the key positions.

Once you are comfortable performing this exercise and you are consistently hitting the desired shapes, you can progress to the exercises to cement the pattern. If you struggle with this exercise, the following two exercises should help you out.

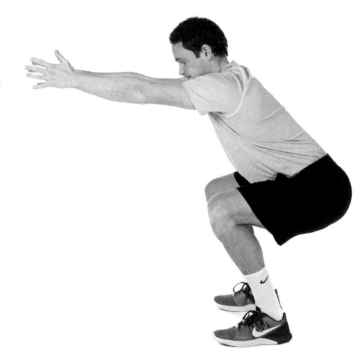

Band around knees squat

A common squatting fault is valgus collapse, where the knees fall inwards. Although the band doesn't physically prevent this from happening, it gives you external feedback to create external rotation torque. This increases muscle activation in the areas that will prevent collapse.

- Place a band around your legs, positioned about 2.5cm above your knees.
- With the hand in position and focusing on maintaining tension on it, perform the body-weight squat with arms in front.

3 x 5 reps of slow lower (4 seconds) with isometric pause (2 seconds) at the bottom of the movement.

Once you are consistently performing this exercise well, go back to the first exercise and see if you're now able to perform it without valgus collapse.

Developing the pattern

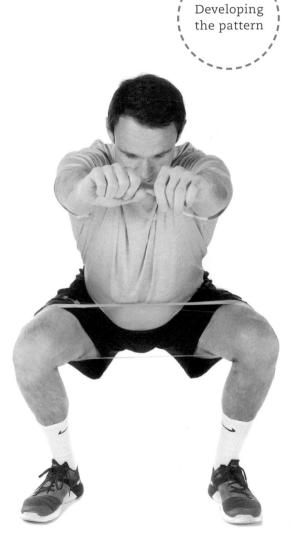

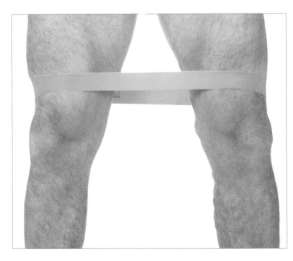

Wall squat

A great exercise for correcting a number of squatting faults, including not getting your hips back, not keeping your shins vertical and excessive flexion of the trunk. A wall squat gives you excellent feedback, even if you're on your own, as your head and knees will get closer to the wall if performed correctly.

Developing the pattern

■ Stand facing a wall and adopt your squat stance with your toes touching the base of the wall or, if you struggle with that, up to 30cm back from it.

■ Place your hands close to the wall, palms facing forwards and at about hip height.

■ Squat down, bringing your hands down, as far as you can go without your head or knees touching the wall or you falling backwards. Don't expect to hit full depth.

■ Pause at the bottom, return to standing and repeat.

The squat can throw up an interesting conundrum. Learning the correct pattern can be difficult without external loading. Some athletes don't get it by doing the drills already described but, once you apply some load, it just seems to click. However, this doesn't mean that, if you're struggling with developing the correct pattern, you should just pile on the load. Bodyweight squatting mastery has to be gained, otherwise there's significant potential for injury. If you feel that some load may help, try the following two exercises with a light load but constantly revisit the previous three exercises to gauge whether the heightened awareness that load should have given you has helped.

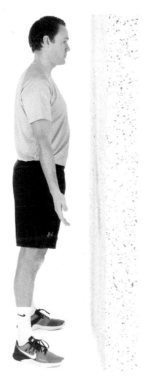

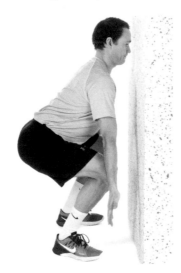

3 x 5 reps of slow lower (4 seconds) with isometric pause (2 seconds) at the bottom of the movement.

Once you are consistently performing this exercise well, go back to the first exercise.

Pick-up squat

Adding some external load in front of the body forces the muscles of the trunk to engage to maintain the positions of the torso and also helps the positioning of the knees.

- Place a dumbbell or kettlebell on the floor between your feet and squat down to pick it up, focusing on the key squat coaching points.
- Keep hold of the load and complete the desired number of repetitions while maintaining the appropriate shape.

Cementing the pattern

Progression 1

3 x 5 reps with a 4-second lower, 2-second pause at the bottom of the movement and controlled lift (7–8 RPE).

Progression 2

3 x 10 reps with a normal smooth land-controlled lifting tempo (7–8 RPE).

You should perform Progression 1 until you are comfortable and confident with the pattern under load as, by slowing the movement down, it allows for more control. Moving on to Progression 2 increases the velocity of the movement.

If you struggle with the range to pick the load off the floor, you can place the dumbbell or kettlebell on a small step or some plates.

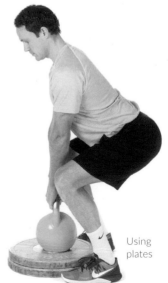

Using plates

CONTROL THROUGH RANGE UNSUPPORTED CORRECTIVE EXERCISES

Goblet squat

Holding the load at chest height increases the centre of mass, therefore challenging the trunk muscle to maintain its position.

■ Hold a dumbbell, kettlebell or plate at chest height.

■ Adopt your strong squat position.

■ Holding the load, complete the desired number of reps, maintaining good form and not allowing it to pull you forwards.

■ If you find under load that your knees are falling inwards, you can use a band as in the band around knees squat on page 119.

Progression 1

3 x 5 reps with a 4-second lower, 2-second pause at the bottom of the movement and controlled lift (7–8 RPE).

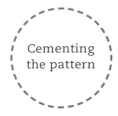

Cementing the pattern

Progression 2

3 x 10 reps with a normal smooth land-controlled lifting tempo (7–8 RPE).

You should perform Progression 1 until you are comfortable and confident with the pattern under load as, by slowing the movement down, it allows for more control. Moving to Progression 2 increases the velocity of the movement.

With these two exercises, you should be able to progress your squatting to a reasonable level and get the movement pattern solidly cemented. However, if you squat regularly, you will find that your grip/upper body strength and the weight of the load you are able to hold in your hands becomes the limiting factor. At that stage, if you're 100 per cent confident in your form, you should consider progressing to the squat variants described in Chapter 5.

How deep is deep enough?

There is much discussion and debate around squat depth. Go to any strength training or bodybuilding forum and you'll see that whether to squat 'arse to grass' or 'thighs just below parallel' divides opinion in the same way as Campagnolo versus Shimano for cyclists. In truth, the answer, like most things, is that it depends on the ability and goals of the individual athlete. There are so many considerations as to what is an appropriate squat depth, going right back to genetics and bone structure. Your hip joint structure will determine to an extent how well you're able to squat. Stuart McGill, a noted spinal researcher, talks about a 'Celtic hip' and a 'Dalmation hip', peculiar to eastern Europeans. He has found that, as a general population, eastern Europeans tend to have shallower hip sockets that facilitate squatting, whereas Celts less so. Squatting is not just about the hip, though; it involves multiple joints interacting together, with the pelvis and lumbar spine also key. Therefore, for such a complex movement and so many individual factors, giving blanket one-size-fits-all advice for depth is both impossible and irresponsible. Ultimately, the most important thing, especially when squatting under load, is the maintenance of a neutral spine while flexing at the hips. This calls for mobility and stability in all the key areas and it's this that should govern squat depth.

▼ *Your genetics, mobility and training goals will determine your appropriate depth of squat.*

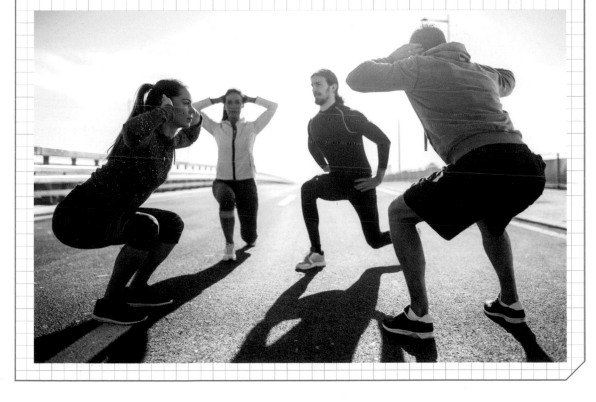

CONTROL THROUGH RANGE UNSUPPORTED: SPLIT SQUAT CORRECTIVES

The split squat takes the mechanics of the squat pattern and places it into an asymmetrical split stance. This is important as, when you think of many of our day-to-day movement patterns, such as walking, running and cycling, we actually perform equally loaded two-footed movements relatively infrequently. As the basics of the hinge and squat have already been established, there is less of an emphasis on patterning and the exercises have more of a training feel straight away. Focusing on getting split squats right is very worthwhile and, requiring far less load to create a training stimulus than two-footed exercises (bodyweight is often sufficient),

they're brilliant for travel routines where equipment availability is minimal.

There are a number of key coaching points to be aware of:

■ Most people perform split squats and their variations with an upright posture. However, if we were to look at our squat position, it is probably very different and therefore represents flawed mechanics.

■ We recommend a forward torso lean posture on to the heel, which loads the muscles of the lower leg more evenly, therefore training it in the manner it was meant to operate.

■ A good split squat should involve solid hinge mechanics, whereas an overly upright posture places greater stress on the knees and low back while minimising stress on the glutes and upper thighs.

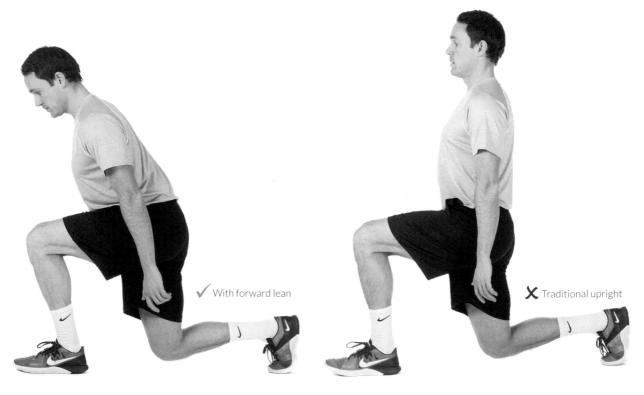

✔ With forward lean

✘ Traditional upright

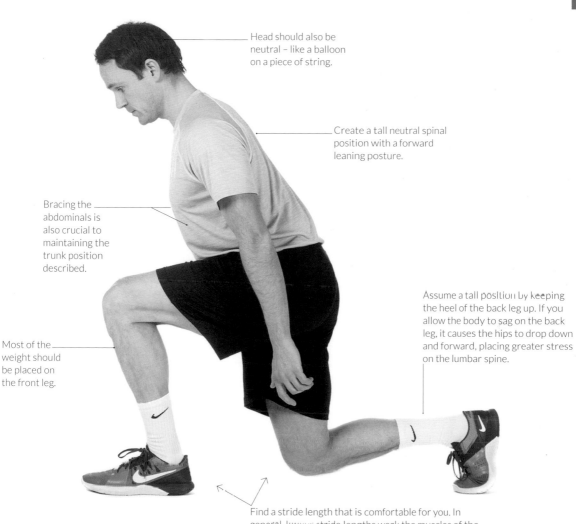

Head should also be neutral – like a balloon on a piece of string.

Create a tall neutral spinal position with a forward leaning posture.

Bracing the abdominals is also crucial to maintaining the trunk position described.

Assume a tall position by keeping the heel of the back leg up. If you allow the body to sag on the back leg, it causes the hips to drop down and forward, placing greater stress on the lumbar spine.

Most of the weight should be placed on the front leg.

Find a stride length that is comfortable for you. In general, longer stride lengths work the muscles of the hip more intensely, while shorter stride lengths work the quadriceps more. The critical thing is that stride length shouldn't dictate mechanics.

■ When initiating the movement, focus on the torso moving straight up and down while maintaining the position described. You don't want horizontal displacement of the torso.

■ Don't drop the knee all the way to the floor – while it is important to work through a full range, dropping the knee to the floor often causes loss of tension in the body and consequently in the position.

■ Initiate the upwards movement by driving the floor away. This should help maintain the required posture on the ascent.

Split squat

The starting place is practising the above coaching points in the split squat as performed in the assessment. When learning the drill, performing slow and controlled descent phases with a pause in the bottom position can really help develop a feel for the movement. It also works the smaller stabilising muscles harder as they have to maintain body position for longer.

Developing and cementing the pattern

■ From a standing position, take an exaggerated step forwards, keeping your feet in line or very slightly offset.

■ As you do so, lift the heel of your rear foot and effectively perform a hip hinge. This creates a forward lean. A common coaching fault for split squats and lunges is to try to maintain an upright torso.

■ Brace your trunk muscles and maintain a neutral spine.

■ By bending both legs at the knees, drop towards the ground. Think of a straight down movement.

■ Keep your front shin vertical and your knee above the midpoint of your foot.

■ You're looking to achieve a 90-degree angle in both your front and rear knee.

■ Return to the start position, maintaining the form points above.

■ If you struggle to get the position described, a half foam roller under the ball of the front foot can help.

To check if you're getting the right position, do the 'Split Squat to Squat Test'. Once you're in the bottom position of your split squat, you should be able to bring your back foot forwards into a regular two-footed squat without adjusting your body position. If you had to change your body position significantly or couldn't do it, your position probably wasn't correct.

Split squat to squat

Walking lunges

A commonly seen and prescribed split squat variation is the walking lunge, but, for the majority of people, it's not an appropriate exercise. This dynamic variation often causes form and mechanics to degrade. There are several reasons for this. Firstly, the walking momentum has a tendency to drive the hips too far forwards, making it difficult to keep optimal hip hinge mechanics. This is why many lifters complain of knee and low back pain associated with lunges. Secondly, the walking or stepping lunge (forward or backward) is much more difficult to correct and fine-tune. The movement occurs too quickly to make subtle adjustments to form. Stationary lunges, particularly when done in a controlled and methodical fashion, allow you to hone in on your mechanics and make adjustments. Finally, many people have poor balance and stability. If you have faulty hip, foot and ankle mechanics, walking lunges set you up for failure and further degradations in technique. You'll be forced to rely on compensation patterns and straddled stance alignment in order to maintain balance. However, once proper lunge technique is mastered and all traces of dysfunction are eliminated, walking lunges can be appropriately programmed and have some unique benefits.

Loaded split squat

The basic split squat can be progressed by loading with external implements, which can be held in a number of ways. Loading, as with other exercises, challenges the neuromuscular system further and therefore provides a greater training effect.

■ Ideally, load by holding dumbbells in your hands as in our experience this helps to encourage good technique.

■ You can use a chest-held dumbbell or kettlebell as with the goblet squat, but ensure you still set the split squat correctly and don't adopt an overly upright posture.

Developing and cementing the pattern

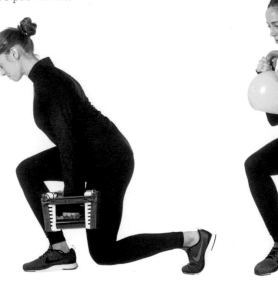
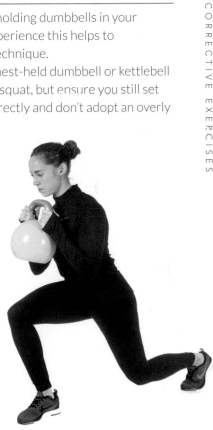

Rear foot elevated squat

Another progression of the split squat is the rear foot elevated squat or, as it's sometimes known, the Bulgarian split squat. Elevating the rear foot forces more load on to the front leg, so increasing the work that the muscles in the front of the leg have to do. This is therefore a good option if you don't have access to implements to load the movement.

■ Technically, the movement is the same as the split squat described previously and you should follow the same coaching points.

■ The key is getting the appropriate elevation of the back leg. Most people tend to go too high, which drives many of the positions we are trying to avoid. The exact box height will depend on many factors such as height, limb length, etc., but should be dictated by your ability to perform the movement correctly. As a general rule of thumb, most people will find their optimal box height to be around 30–40cm.

■ Once the movement has been mastered, it can be loaded, ideally using dumbbells in the hands.

For these three exercises, when first learning the movements, perform 3 x 5 reps with a 4-second lower, 2-second pause at the bottom of the movement and controlled lift (7–8 RPE).

Once proficient with this, a more dynamic sets and reps scheme can be used: 3 x 10 reps with a normal smooth land-controlled lifting tempo (7–8 RPE).

Developing and cementing the pattern

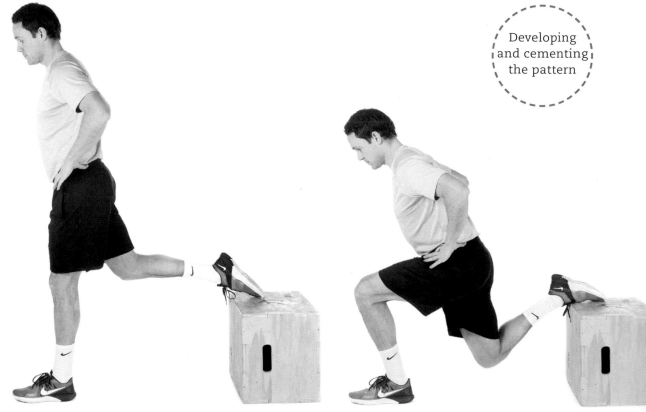

THORACIC SPINE

CONTROL THROUGH RANGE UNSUPPORTED: PRESS-UP CORRECTIVES

The humble press-up is a much underrated exercise and many gym-goers will tend to abandon it fairly early in their lifting career and instead move on to the bench press and its various iterations. However, especially if significant upper body size gains aren't a goal, the press-up is an extremely useful exercise that offers many benefits when performed correctly.

The abdominal muscles have a significant role in stabilising the spine during a press-up, making it a highly time-effective exercise as it can negate the need for specific abdominal exercises.

It is a closed chain exercise, with the hands and feet 'locked' in place on the floor, which forces the upper body to work in harmony, in contrast to open chain supported exercises, which can cause issues for some people.

It can easily be modified to overload different muscles of the trunk and upper body. For example, press-ups with one hand on a medicine ball pose a significant challenge for the abdominals, while a clapping press-up is a real test of the explosive strength of your chest, arms and shoulders.

It can be performed anywhere with no equipment needed.

▼ *An age-old exercise that if done properly is incredibly effective and versatile.*

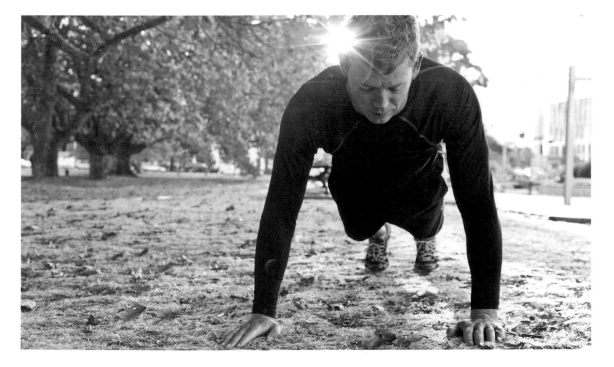

Common Press-up Problems

If you have struggled with the press-up in the assessment or have simply never been able to manage one, it's likely that you're experiencing problems with one or both of two areas.

If viewed from above, the arms and trunk form a T rather than an arrowhead. This is problematic as it causes unusual loading patterns in the shoulders, especially at the bottom of the movement, which can lead to pain and inflammation.

Your hips tend to sag during the movement, which causes an inappropriate load to be placed on the spine. This is usually due to a lack of awareness of trunk positioning and/or the strength to stabilise it.

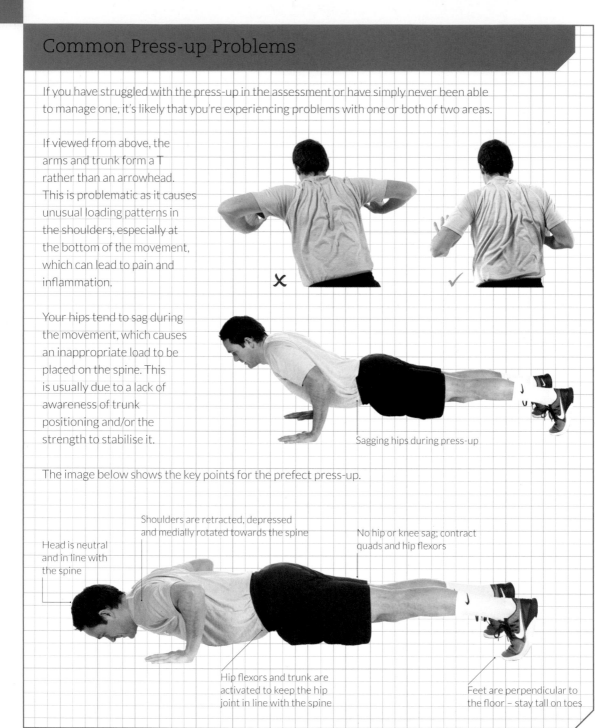

Sagging hips during press-up

The image below shows the key points for the prefect press-up.

Shoulders are retracted, depressed and medially rotated towards the spine

No hip or knee sag; contract quads and hip flexors

Head is neutral and in line with the spine

Hip flexors and trunk are activated to keep the hip joint in line with the spine

Feet are perpendicular to the floor – stay tall on toes

Press-up plank

The press-up plank teaches proper whole body alignment and strengthens the musculature involved in holding a straight and strong press-up position.

Developing and cementing the pattern

- Adopt an 'up' press-up position, ensuring you follow all of the key coaching points.
- Hold the position for the times given or until you can no longer maintain good form.
- Try placing a foam roller under your feet, as this forces you into optimal alignment.

Aim to build up progressively to a 2-minute hold.

To train your capacity to achieve this if unable to initially, perform 2–3 sets of 30–60 seconds with short 30-second rests in between. Test regularly for your maximum hold and adjust time accordingly but ensure that you only hold until loss of good form.

CONTROL THROUGH RANGE UNSUPPORTED CORRECTIVE EXERCISES

Incline press-up

Developing
and cementing
the pattern

As we discussed during the assessment, an incline press-up provides a far better press-up modification than pivoting on the knees, which doesn't develop the correct alignment or movement pattern. Once you have worked on proper alignment with the press-up plank, even if you lack the strength and control for a full press-up, you can use this exercise to start developing the movement pattern.

■ Adopt a press-up position with your hands on a box, step or stair.

■ The higher the object, the less 'load' you'll be lifting. Experiment with the height of object that works best for your ability.

■ Lower yourself down, maintaining correct alignment, and then think about pressing the object away from you to return to the start position.

3 x 10 reps. Once you can manage this, you can start to reduce the height of the object and, in doing so, progress towards the full movement.

Negative press-up (with band assistance)

Once the position and pattern have been developed, it's time to start working from the floor. You can use this exercise in conjunction with the previous two exercises so that you're developing both the strength and movement pattern for a full press-up in conjunction with each other.

The banded version of the exercise with a partner serves two purposes. It gives proprioceptive feedback of trunk position and you can also get your partner to provide assistance to allow you to complete the lifting phase of the movement.

Developing and cementing the pattern

■ Adopt the 'up' press-up position, as if performing a press-up plank.
■ Under full control and maintaining alignment, lower yourself down to the floor.
■ Put your knees down, return to the start position and repeat.
■ If you're working with a partner, get them to stand above you holding a band around your hips.

3 x 10 reps.

Full press-up

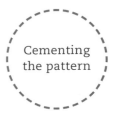

Cementing the pattern

Working through the previous exercises, you'll know when you're ready to move on to a full press-up.

■ Start in the 'up' position with your hands on the floor.

■ Before lowering, scan through the coaching points to ensure correct alignment.

■ Lower under control so that your chest is approximately a fist's distance from the floor.

■ Maintaining alignment, press away from the floor to return to the start position.

■ Repeat.

Aim to complete 3 x 10 reps.

Even if you can only manage a single rep, do that and then use negative press-ups or incline press-ups to complete the set. Try to add an additional 'full rep' each session.

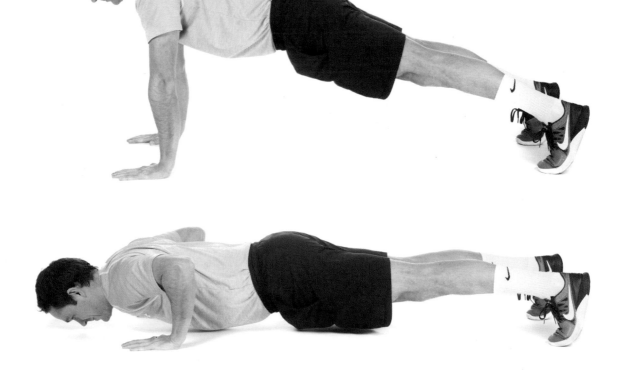

CONTROL THROUGH RANGE UNSUPPORTED (OPTIONAL): INVERTED ROW CORRECTIVES

The inverted row is a great exercise for building upper back strength and can help alleviate some of the postural issues that cyclists face. If performed correctly, it can be similar to the press-up, helping with developing the stability of the trunk and the posterior chain. It works well with the press-up as it trains the antagonist muscle groups.

It is essentially the same mechanics as a press-up and many of the same cues apply, but the body moves in the opposite direction. We have found, though, that it is often easier to learn these mechanics with the press-up before progressing to the inverted row.

In order to perform an inverted row, you will need some kind of suspension training device (e.g. TRX) or a bar in a rack. For this reason, it's an optional step in the assessment but if you are able to accommodate it, it's well worth the effort. Similar to the squat and the split squat, if you have press-up mechanics nailed, then progressing to the inverted row shouldn't be too much of an issue. Therefore, the corrective exercises are fewer in number and will definitely feel like training.

For all the inverted row variations, it's important to avoid extreme pulling positions. Many people over-pull, thinking that's better, but it can lead to problems. It causes the head of the humerus to glide forward and create unwanted movement at the shoulder joint, which can cause inflammation and ultimately pain. When performing any pulling movement, it's essential to maintain proper alignment of the shoulder joint.

Scaled inverted row

Just as we elevated your upper body to change the angle of the press-up and make it more manageable, you can do the same for the inverted row. The nearer your body is to horizontal, the more difficult it is.

■ Set up for an inverted row, looking for a body position of approximately 45 degrees.
■ Work at this body angle, aiming for 10 reps at 7–8 RPE.
■ Once you can manage this for 3 sets, lower yourself and work back through the process.
■ Placing a foam roller under the back of the ankles can aid in attaining and maintaining the correct body position as it forces dorsiflexion of the foot, which engages the entire anterior chain.

The end point of the Scaled Inverted Row progression is 3 x 10 reps at 7–8 RPE of the Inverted Row as described in the assessment.

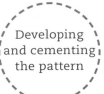

Developing and cementing the pattern

45 degree angle

With foam roller

Feet elevated inverted row

Increase the difficulty of the movement by elevating the feet.

■ Use a box or step to elevate your feet.
■ Ensure you maintain form and a strong body position.

Aim for 3 x 10 reps at 7–8 RPE.

Cementing the pattern

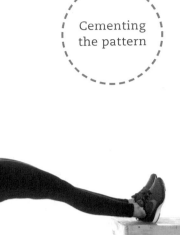

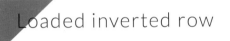

Loaded inverted row

Progress from the previous exercise by adding load. This challenges both the trunk muscles and the upper back to maintain position and pull to the desired position.

■ Set up in the same way as above but with a weight plate on your abdomen.
■ Maintain form and position without allowing the load to pull your midsection towards the ground.

Aim for 3 x 10 reps at 7–8 RPE and then up the load.

Cementing the pattern

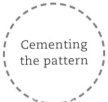

Aero gains 2

In Chapter 1 we discussed how, by working on your range of movement, you'd improve your ability to attain a more aerodynamic position on the bike. At this stage in the plan, and moving on to the more advanced and loaded exercises in Chapter 5, you'll compound these gains by developing the strength to hold this position and to provide a stable platform from which to deliver power to your pedals.

In the first aero gains discussion box, we outlined the significant role of being able to rotate your pelvis forward to achieve a good flat back position on the bike. Achieving this flatter back position is only part way there, though, as you also need to be able to hold it. Key exercises to achieving this will be improving overall glute strength to maintain a stable hip position on your pelvis as well as developing good trunk strength and stability by working on planks and side planks.

Good shoulder range needs to be supported by some control and strength for the neck to extend effectively. This facilitates both seeing up the road and maintaining whatever is the best aero head shrug/tuck for your riding position. Also, the shoulders are the base off which you load, when down in an aero position. With often relatively poor upper body conditioning, this is nearly always a limitation in cyclists. You see the results of poor conditioning in the shoulder and triceps through poor head stability, neck pain and constant movement out of position to relieve tightness or aching. Every time you move your head or come out of your aero position, you're losing time. A weak upper body will have a knock-on effect all the way back to the engine house of the glutes and hips. With your upper body fatiguing and unable to hold position, you'll find yourself shifting back and forwards in the saddle as you try to relieve pressure on your arms and shoulders. Every shift means lost power. Planking movements along with the press-up and inverted row progressions will all significantly improve your upper body strength.

Because an aero position is a static supported position, you will be making significant progress as you work through the control through range supported corrective exercises. Moving on to control through range unsupported corrective exercises, such as squats, will definitely condition key joints and muscles involved in holding your aero position but it's important not to neglect actually riding in the position to develop your tolerance and adaptation to it. If you find you haven't or can't get to the control through range unsupported corrective exercises, keep working on the more supported exercises. These will still transfer well to the bike and yield gains.

▼ *Strengthening and improving upper body and trunk mobility will allow you to hold a more aero position.*

Scheduling

As the exercises at this level are much more like actual training and we start to introduce load, more thought and a different approach to scheduling has to be taken. It's possible that this level of off the bike training could have an acute negative effect on your ability to perform cycling workouts and, vice versa, your cycling could impact on your off the bike gains. Follow the guidelines laid out at the beginning of this chapter and schedule focused off the bike training blocks into periods of the year when cycle training is reduced or at lower intensity.

RPE

Rather than using percentage of maximal lifts, which can be dangerous and inaccurate for most non-specialist lifters, we use a simple RPE scale. As well as providing an accurate and personalised way to determine sets and reps, it encourages the exerciser to develop a higher level of body awareness.

Squatting

Pick up almost any cycling training book with a strength routine and you can guarantee it will contain squats. There's no doubting their effectiveness as an exercise, but hopefully, in having worked through this book, you'll now appreciate their complexity and that, for the vast majority of cyclists, going to the gym, loading up a barbell and squatting is a recipe for disaster. As you reach this stage in the plan, take time working on the squat progressions and don't rush to load the movement until you're 100 per cent confident you're doing it right.

CHAPTER 5

TAKING IT FURTHER

If you have worked successfully through the assessment using the corrective exercises and are regularly performing the top tier exercises in Chapter 4, you've reached an excellent level of conditioning above and beyond that of even many elite riders.

If you want to carry on progressing your off the bike conditioning, this chapter outlines how to construct a more advanced training plan and gives some suggestions for exercises to include. Even if you're not yet at this stage with your off the bike training, you should still read through this chapter as it will give you valuable information regarding programming and session structure.

If you haven't reached this level, don't worry or beat yourself up, just keep up the work that you're doing. The fact is that cycling, daily life, genetics and injury conspire to limit full movement patterns and there are

movements that some riders will always struggle with. Even if you hit a plateau at the lower level of corrective exercises, simply by maintaining that ability and continuing to focus on your areas of weakness, you'll be improving both on the bike and your robustness off it. Again, this brings us back to one of the earliest and key points of this book: any off the bike conditioning has to be uniquely tailored to the needs of the individual rider.

▼ *Many pro riders don't achieve this level of conditioning and you don't necessarily need to progress to the exercises in this chapter to be a highly successful and healthy rider.*

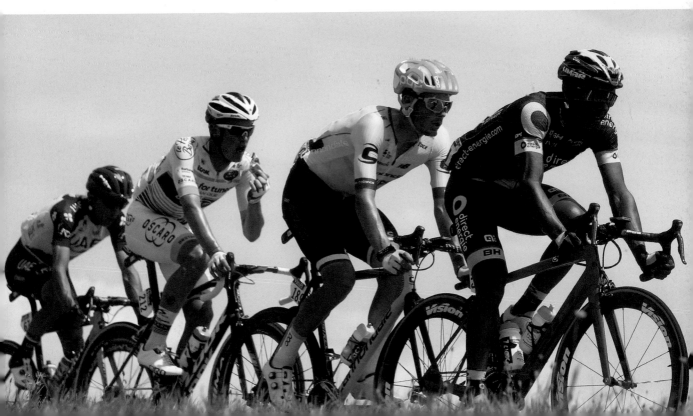

CONSTRUCTING A PLAN

We have already given some guidelines about scheduling your off the bike training in Chapter 4. With some of those exercises delivering significant training load, how they affect and interact with your on the bike performance and training has to be considered. As you progress through the top tier of corrective exercises and on to the more advanced options suggested in this chapter, it's necessary to have a more structured approach to how your off the bike work fits into your overall training plan.

Developing a detailed training plan is a time-intensive but extremely valuable process to go through as, by setting goals and expectations for specific blocks of training, you can minimise interference between on and off the bike work and maximise gains. Committing pen to paper and determining focused training blocks can be a powerful tool to improving your performance. While a highly detailed explanation of training planning is beyond the scope of this book by following some relatively simple guidelines you should be able to construct a plan to optimise your training time. It's worth remembering that, although planning is important, it's no substitute for actually doing the training! Many of us will have procrastinated and put off revising for exams at school by producing elaborate revision timetables. Don't do the same with your training.

WHAT IT TAKES

The first thing to consider is what you're trying to achieve and what you'll need to do to make this happen. Within the Great Britain Cycling Team, the question 'what will it take to win?' is at the heart of everything we do. Once we've identified a target, such as gold in the team pursuit, we work out what time the riders would have to achieve and, from that, the power they'll need to produce to achieve this. We'll then look at how much time we have to get there. It's then a case of working back from this target and producing a training plan that will elevate the team to where they need to be. Once you've identified your main targets for the year, do the same thing. As a general rule of thumb, it takes around 8–12 weeks to make any real changes in your physical attributes. Therefore, where possible, blocks of focus and work should be planned with this in mind.

YOUR TRAINING YEAR

The TASMT, stretching and, to an extent, developing the pattern exercises can be performed year-round and shouldn't cause much fatigue or impact significantly on your cycling performance. You can therefore continue to work on these exercises throughout the season and around key events. However, the more demanding training exercises, in the upper tier of Chapter 4 and this chapter, need to be focused on during periods of the year when cycling performance is less important, such as the off season.

LEADING IN TO EVENTS

In the same way as you'll taper your cycling training down in the lead-up to a big event, it's also necessary to do the same with your off the bike training. The reduction in training volume typically begins 14–28 days prior to competition. The exact length and nature of an athlete's taper is dependent on a number of factors, is highly personal and can often be a case of trial and error. However, it's normal to cease any loaded strength training 7–10 days prior to competition.

A taper into competition for someone performing 2 sessions per week may look like this:

■ 3 weeks out, reduce strength training sessions to 1 per week. This is a 50 per cent reduction in load, which is in line with research in this area. Intensity should at least be maintained and possibly increased (i.e. try to lift the same load or more).
■ 2 weeks out, strength training volume could be reduced further by dropping from 3 sets per exercise to 2 sets.
■ 1 week out, no strength sessions are performed.

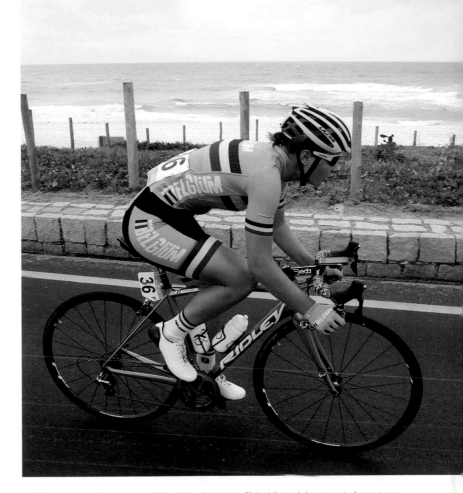

▲ In the lead up to key events, you'll need to adapt your off the bike training as part of your taper.

As we've already mentioned, this is very individual, so after the event it's important to reflect on your performance and the factors that have contributed to it, and then to adjust your plan for your next events accordingly.

Once you have a rough overall plan of your year divided into appropriate 8–12-week blocks, you can start to map out the detail of the phases of training, determining the focus of both on and off the bike training.

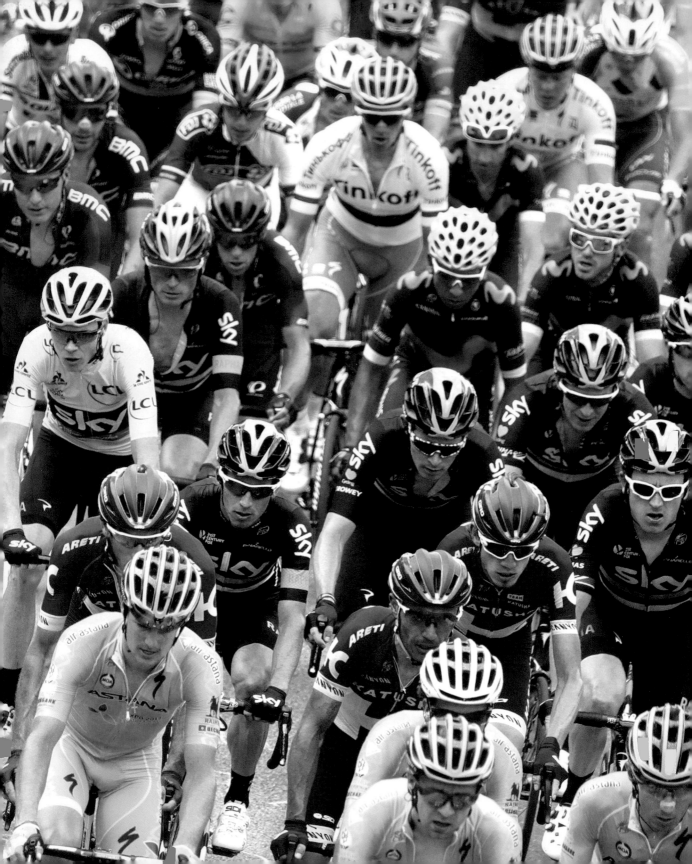

There are many ways of doing this but the key thing is that it makes sense to you and you believe in your plan. A good guideline is to start with more general conditioning and increase in specificity the closer you get to the event. For example, if you have 6 sessions in a week, you may begin for the first 3 weeks of a block with an even split of 3 cycling workouts and 3 dedicated strength sessions. This could then change to a 2 and 4 split in favour of cycling and, as the event gets nearer and you taper down both on and off the bike work, a 1 and 3 split. Depending on the event, the emphasis of work along with the volume would also change through the block. For example, if targeting a time trial, the on the bike training would transition from general conditioning on the road bike to harder race intensity efforts on the time trial bike. This would sit well with the reduction in off the bike training as that work wouldn't negatively interfere with the demanding cycling workouts. This process of first laying down the general foundations of fitness and conditioning and then focusing in on the specific demands of particular events should be a constant theme in your training. A good analogy is building a house. No matter how impressive the top floors and roof look, unless the foundations are solid, that house is coming down.

◄ *Lay solid foundations of general conditioning and then focus on the specific demands of events.*

PLANNING YOUR WEEK AND STRUCTURING SESSIONS

Having worked through to this stage of the book, you'll already be very familiar with the assessment and how you should be continuously referring to it, retesting and determining the areas that you need to target. Even once you have 'passed' every test, it's more than likely that an especially hard day on the bike, a long drive or a host of other factors could cause part of your body to demand some corrective work. You may even find that to be able to perform some of the more advanced exercises correctly, you need to work through some corrective exercises in a preparation for lifting routine.

Guidelines for daily sessions

You should also look to continue to include on a daily basis the corrective exercises that are most appropriate to you. These only have to be bite-sized sessions, as consistency is the key.

- Can be micro sessions performed frequently throughout the day.
- Can also include one dedicated longer session, depending on schedule.
- Will largely comprise TASMT and stretching exercises.
- Pick the low-hanging fruit from the assessment (i.e. the exercises that you've found have the biggest impact on you).
- Work through the activities and continually reassess to check whether you're making a change.
- The exercises you do can vary from day to day.

■ Can be performed pre-training or post-training or at any time throughout the day, even in front of the TV in the evening!

Guidelines for strength sessions

In Chapter 4 we laid out a number of guidelines for how to incorporate sessions with more demanding training exercises into your routine. As these exercises become more advanced, greater loads are added and the focus shifts to genuine strength gains and the guidelines for strength sessions can be expanded on.

■ Perform 2–3 sessions per week (depending on focus of training block, time of year and closeness to competition).
■ Ensure 48 hours between sessions.
■ Refer to the guidelines in Chapter 4 for minimising the interference between endurance and resistance training.
■ Each session would ideally include a hinge, a squat/split squat, a push, a pull and ideally a trunk movement.
■ Pick the exercises that are appropriate to you – don't just go for all of the most advanced options.
■ You may have to schedule time into the session for corrective TASMT and stretching exercises to allow you to be able to perform an exercise.
■ You might not be at the same level for all exercises or body areas. For example, you may be loading the squat and hinge but still patterning the press-up and inverted row. This isn't an issue; it can be accommodated in your sessions and will constantly change and fluctuate.

Session structure

Each session should ideally consist of hinge, squat or split squat, press, pull and, if you have time, a trunk movement.

Place the exercises you find the most difficult first as this will allow you to focus more resource into that exercise. As well as prioritising your personal weaknesses, which is where you stand to make the greatest gains, you'll have less overall physical and mental fatigue for the movements that you find most challenging.

For example, someone who struggles with hinge and press-up could do:

1 Loaded hinge
2 Press-up
3 Goblet squat
4 Inverted row

Alternatively, for someone who struggles with squat and row it could look like this:

1 Goblet squat
2 Inverted row
3 Loaded hinge
4 Press-up

Use the RPE scale to guide load selection; RPE should remain in the 7–8 range. As you get stronger, loads become heavier to keep you working in that effort range. Remember, it's not just completing a given set with a load that's important, it's doing so with good form.

Recovery between exercises is an important factor but often poorly implemented in training programmes. Endurance athletes often struggle with the concept of rest, thinking that it's always best to try to pack as much into any training session as possible. As a general rule, you should allow enough rest to complete the next set with maximum effort and quality. For the purposes of developing strength, this is typically 2–3 minutes between sets of the same exercise. However, as you get stronger you may need to rest longer than this in order to maintain the level of effort. Some elite track sprint cyclists have been known to rest at least 5 minutes between sets of heavy squats.

The downside of this, particularly if you aren't a professional athlete with all day to train, is that sessions can take a long time. One way to manage this is to perform sets of

an exercise that stresses a different part of the body – for example, a squat and an inverted row tend to work well together, while a hinge and press-up also tend to fit well. In this situation, you can still complete training at a good level while also making it more time-effective – for example, you could perform a set of a squat exercise then rest 90 seconds before performing a set of inverted row followed by another 90 seconds' rest. You manage the overall session time and the fatigue much more effectively by preserving the rest between sets of the same exercise.

Once you are able to perform the top-tier exercises described in Chapter 4 with a decent level of load, you have options as to how to progress your training and vary your routine. The first option is to stick with those same

▼ Adequate rest between exercises is as important as the sets and reps – something that endurance athletes often forget!

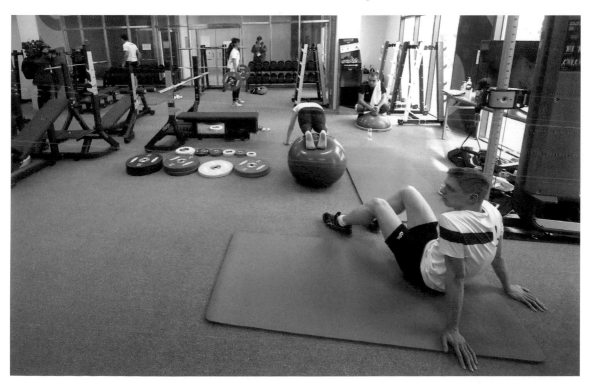

exercises and to simply manipulate intensity and volume. The second option is to progress to some of the more advanced variations described below.

There is no right or wrong. Our general philosophy is to maximise the basics so, nine times out of ten, we would go with the first option. However, there may be situations where this isn't appropriate and you'll want to include or substitute in some alternative exercises. You may only have access to a certain amount of load or find, when squatting for example, that your leg strength outstrips the load you can hold in your hands. Also, you might just want to include a bit more variety in your training.

Set and rep numbers

In Chapter 4, a two-step progression in set and rep number and lifting tempo was given for a number of the exercises:

3 × 5 reps with a 4-second lower, 2-second pause at the bottom of the movement and controlled lift (7–8 RPE).

3 × 10 reps with a normal smooth land-controlled lifting tempo (7–8 RPE).

This is also generally applicable for the advanced exercise options described in this chapter and, unless you have reached a point where you're no longer progressing by increasing load within this structure, there's no need to alter it.

Once you have maxed out your progression on this relatively simplistic rep scheme, it is appropriate to start manipulating the volume and load of sessions in order to continue your strength training gains. One method of doing this is to organise training into periods of higher volume with lower load and lower volume with higher load. This adheres to key training principles such as progression and overload and is well supported in the research.

The basic approach is to work in 3-week phases where you work in a certain set and rep range and then you slightly reduce the volume while increasing the load. An example of this is given below. Obviously, as the reps decrease, the load needs to increase accordingly to keep it in the desired RPE range of 7–8.

Weeks 1–3:	3 × 10
Weeks 4–6:	3 × 8
Weeks 7–9:	3 × 6
Weeks 10–12:	3 × 4

Another iteration of this could use a slightly different strategy where, rather than a progressive reduction in rep number and corresponding increase in load, you go through a bigger variation from one 3-week phase to the next. We have found this to be useful for athletes who have a greater depth of experience of strength training and seem to respond well to the greater amount of variation.

Weeks 1–3:	3 × 10
Weeks 4–6:	3 × 6
Weeks 7–9:	3 × 8
Weeks 10–12:	3 × 4

▶ *Time spent on off the bike conditioning will translate to enhanced comfort, performance and enjoyment when you do get out and ride.*

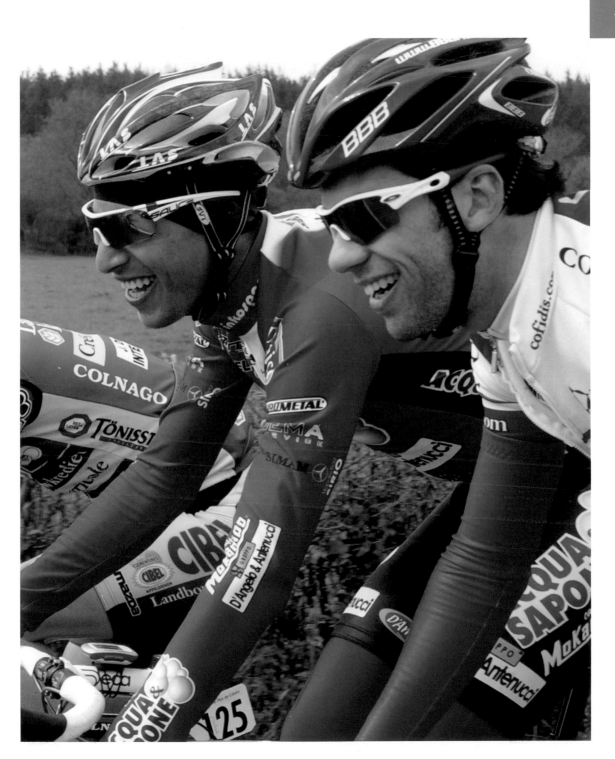

ADVANCED EXERCISES

By no means extensive, these exercise options are suitable progressions and variations to the upper-tier control through range unsupported exercises. Use the set and rep structure described previously unless otherwise noted.

If the movement is unilateral, such as the single leg hinge, single arm row or side plank, perform on each side and then rest.

HINGE

Split stance hinge

A split stance hinge is a simple progression that increases the load on one leg and also increases the stabilisation demand of the exercise at the hip and trunk. It is a good option for those who have mastered the bilateral hinge but aren't ready to load the single leg hinge significantly. If the amount of load used decreases too much, you may actually detrain, so be sure to still include a regular hinge in your routine.

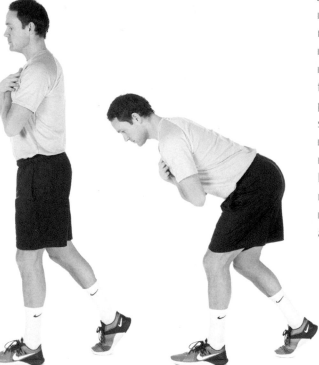

- Set up for a regular hip hinge.
- Step one foot back.
- Unload the rear foot so that it's only providing some stability.
- Hip hinge as normal, aiming to load the front leg as much as possible.
- Change legs and repeat.

Single leg hinge

The single leg hinge is a challenging but important exercise to master. It is performed just like any other hinge but on one leg, which increases the load placed on the stance leg and also helps strengthen the foot and ankle complex.

- Set up for a split stance hinge but completely elevate the rear leg behind you.
- Don't try to keep your rear leg straight, look for a 90-degree bend.
- Avoid pushing for too much range of movement – only go as far as good form and spinal positioning allows.
- Aid maintenance of spinal position by engaging your lats and pinning your shoulders back.
- If holding weights do not let them or your rear foot touch the ground between reps.

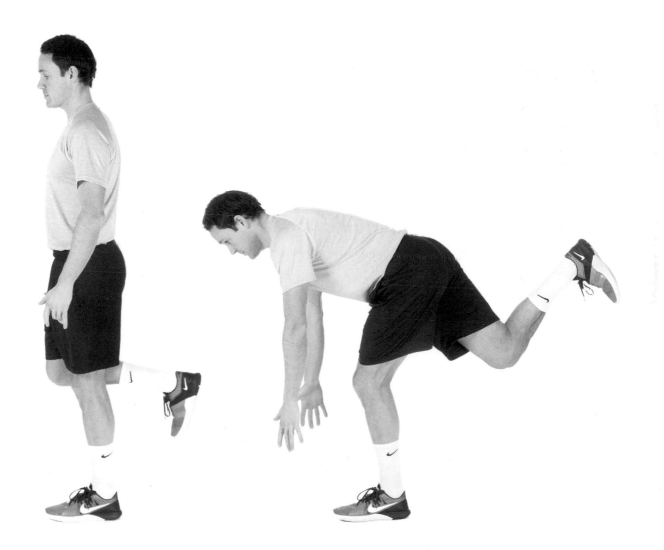

Kettlebell swing

Increasing the speed of movement challenges the hinge pattern in a different way to just increasing the load or reducing the base of support as it forces muscles around the hip and trunk to work in a more reflexive manner, which is quite often more relevant to sporting actions. The swing is a hinge that is performed dynamically. It works best with kettlebells, but dumbbells or plates with handles can also be used.

- Place a kettlebell on the floor between your feet and, with feet hip-width apart, squat down to pick it up.
- Hinge forwards, allowing the kettlebell to swing back between your legs and your weight to shift back on to your heels.
- Drive up from the hinge explosively, allowing the kettlebell to swing to shoulder height.
- At the top of the movement, brace and control the kettlebell as it swings back down and you return into a hinge.

For this exercise, the slow tempo 3 x 5 set/rep sequence doesn't apply, so perform 3 x 10.

SQUAT/SPLIT SQUAT

Kettlebell/dumbbell squat with band

Pretty much any of the squat exercises (including the split squat variations) can be loaded further with the use of a looped band (the same type as you would use for assisted stretching). There are a number of benefits to using a band, the primary benefit being that you can increase the load with minimal equipment. In our experience, the band actually facilitates the execution of the exercise as it also forces you to keep working until the end of the movement because the load increases as you stand up. In addition, this variation could be used in the lead-up to competition as it unloads the bottom position, so has less potential to cause muscle soreness, while preserving the strength benefits through the rest of the range of motion.

- Loop the band around your foot (split squat) or feet (squat) and upper traps/back.
- Perform the movement as normal.

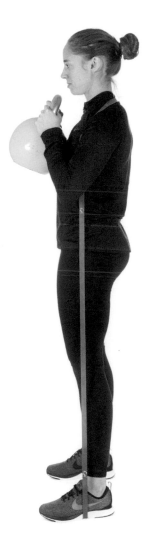
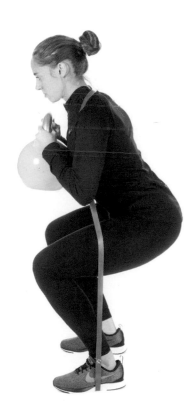

Front rack kettlebell squat

The front rack kettlebell squat is a great way to increase the loading while also maintaining the postural benefits of the goblet squat. By holding a kettlebell and supporting the load on your shoulders, it allows more load to be handled, allowing further leg strengthening.

- Select a kettlebell that you're able to lift to shoulder height or have a training partner help you.
- The body of the kettlebell should rest on your forearm, biceps and shoulder. Your wrist should remain neutral and your fingers should be interlocked.
- Once positioned, squat as normal.

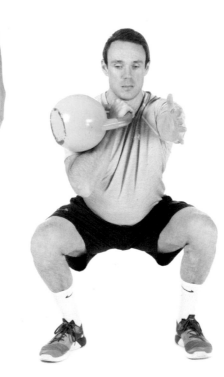

LUNGE VARIATIONS

Lunge variations are progressions of split squat exercises. These challenge your ability to accept impact forces and control the body. In our experience, the reverse lunge is easier to learn first as people seem to hold the posture better, whereas the forward lunge requires the ability to decelerate and then re-accelerate the body. This can be quite challenging for some. We would advise that these exercises are learned with bodyweight only first, then the loading can be gradually progressed. If in doubt about form or positioning, refer back to the split squat correctives in Chapter 4.

Generally, we would start with 'broken' reps, with a slow lower, pause and return. This allows a greater feel for position and makes it more likely that the movement is performed correctly. After this, you should progress the speed and then finally add external loading.

Reverse lunge

In this lunge variation, you step backwards to attain a split squat stance and then lower yourself down to complete the split squat. You then drive out of the bottom position in order to return to the starting position.

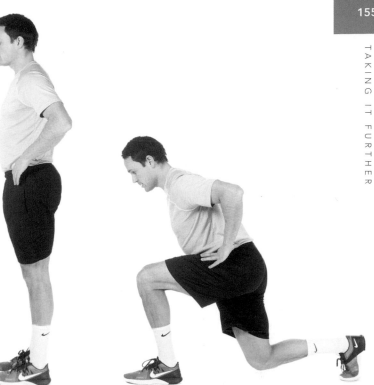

Forward lunge

This is performed as per the reverse lunge but you step forward as opposed to backwards.

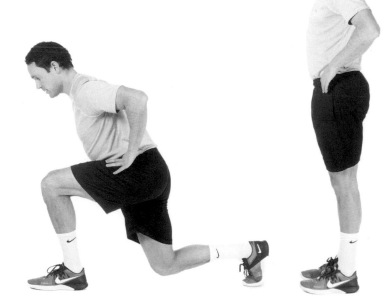

PUSH

There are many options to challenge the upper body pressing muscles. I prefer bodyweight exercise variations, as opposed to barbell or machine bench and chest press, due to the associated benefits of increased trunk stability and shoulder stability mentioned previously.

Loaded press-up

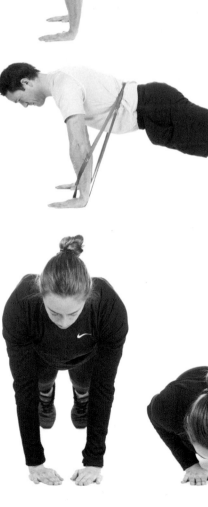

Adding load to a press-up is a great way to increase the training stress on both the upper body muscles and the trunk muscles. This can be done by adding a plate to the back or by using a band.

■ If using plates, they should be placed down towards your hips and lower back. This prevents restriction of your shoulder joint, which can occur if weight is placed too high, and it challenges your trunk more.
■ Similarly, if using a band, it should go around your mid/lower back rather than your upper back/shoulders.

Close grip press-up

This press-up variation increases the load on the triceps.

■ Set up as for a normal press-up but have your hands inside shoulder-width.

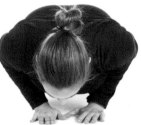

Archer press-up

By adopting an asymmetric hand position,
the load on one arm is significantly increased.
This is a progression towards single-arm
press-ups, a very difficult exercise that
massively challenges both upper body
and trunk strength.

- Set up for a normal press-up and then
straighten one arm out to the side.
- You will probably also have to widen your
foot position.
- Perform the press-up, using the outstretched
arm as little as possible in the movement.
- As you get stronger, elevate the outstretched
arm to progress to a single-arm press-up.

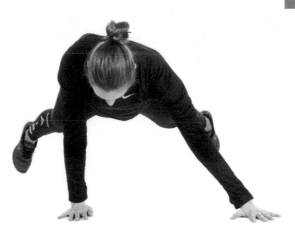

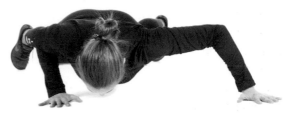

Leg off press-up

Another press-up variation that increases
the stability demand on the trunk.

- Perform a regular press-up but either keep
one leg elevated throughout the set or alternate
legs each rep.

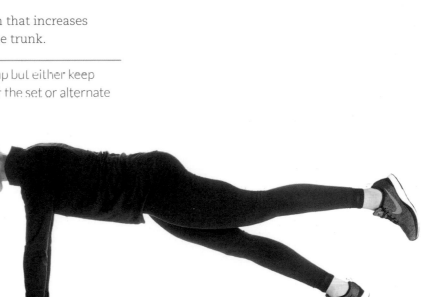

Spiderman press-up

A progression of the leg off press-up that further challenges the lateral stability and control of the trunk.

- Perform a regular press-up but, as the lowering phase of the movement is completed, one leg is brought out to the side.
- Alternate legs each rep.

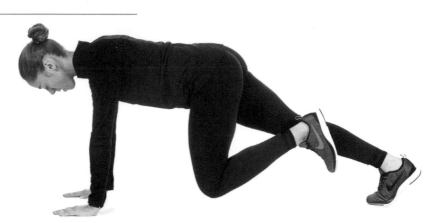

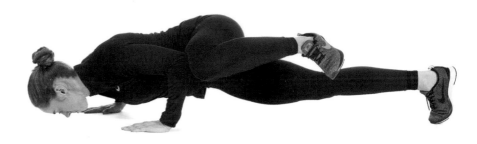

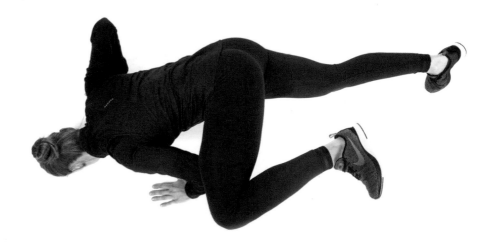

PULL

Single-arm suspension trainer rows

As with other single limb variations, the single-arm suspension trainer row increases the amount of trunk stabilisation that is required so essentially provides more bang for your buck. In addition to this, it increases the shoulder stabilisation demand.

- Use either a suspension system or a bar secured at hip height on a Smith machine or power rack.
- Hold the bar with an overhand grip and bend your knees to 90 degrees with your feet flat on the floor.
- Make sure your body forms a straight line from your knees to your shoulders.
- Release one hand, bracing so as not to rotate away from the bar, and hold it straight up.
- Keeping your body rigid, pull your chest towards the bar, lower and repeat.
- Progress by straightening your legs.

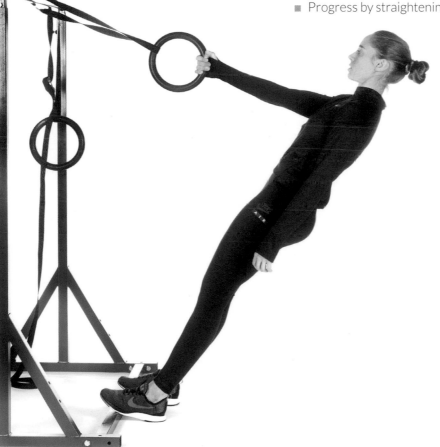

Pull-ups

If you have mastered the horizontal pulling exercises described, you are ready to attack pull-ups. Be warned, though – pull-ups are a significantly harder exercise and, for some, attaining a good level of proficiency at pull-ups can take quite a while. It is, however, a great exercise for strengthening the upper body pulling muscles and, if performed correctly, can also be a potent stimulus for the trunk.

You can grip the handle in many different ways: palm forward, palm backwards or palms facing each other. The muscle recruitment doesn't change significantly enough to say that one way is better than another, so we generally suggest mixing up the grips regularly and becoming strong in all positions.

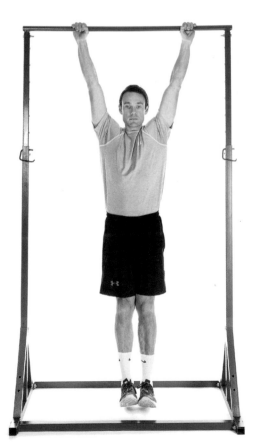
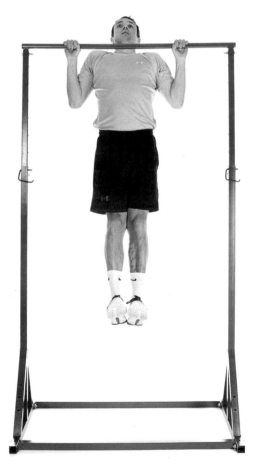

■ No matter what grip you use, it's essential that the pull-up is slow and controlled, with no swinging or 'kipping' involved.

■ Keep your legs straight and then dorsiflex your feet, dropping your heels and bringing your toes towards your shins.

■ Pull strongly, bringing your chest towards the bar.

■ On your first couple of attempts you may struggle to complete a full set or even a single rep, so some kind of regression is necessary. A simple way to reduce the load is by using a band to assist you in the lifting phase of the movement.

■ Once you are proficient with pull-ups, load can be added in a number of ways, although a dumbbell at your feet is probably the easiest. Loading in this way helps reinforce mechanics at the same time as strengthening the upper body musculature.

TRUNK

Static side plank

Similar to a plank, the side plank hold develops the endurance capabilities of the trunk muscles. The side plank develops the lateral component of the trunk.

- Start on your side with your feet together and one forearm directly below your shoulder.
- Brace your trunk and raise your hips off the ground until your body is in a straight line from head to feet. All your weight will be on your elbow and the outside of your bottom foot.
- Hold the position without letting your hips drop or rotating backwards or forwards.
- Aim to build up progressively to a 90-second hold each side.

If you are initially unable to achieve a 90-second hold, perform 2–3 sets of 30–60 seconds with short 30-second rests in between. Test regularly for your maximum hold and adjust time accordingly, but ensure that you only hold until loss of good form.

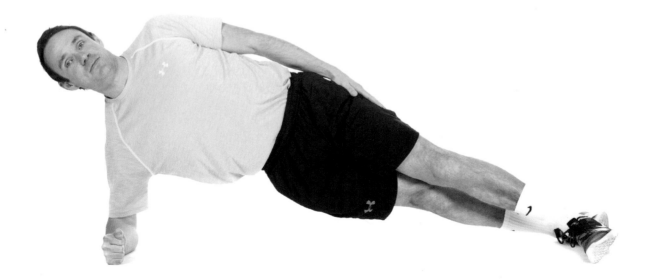

Dynamic side planks

Dynamic side planks are a progression that can be used to train the reactive capabilities of the trunk (i.e. the ability to stabilise while performing a movement). There are many options here, but our two preferred options are below.

Side plank snatch

- Set up for a regular side plank but hold a dumbbell in your upper hand.
- Snatch the dumbbell explosively to a position directly over your shoulder by pulling your flexed elbow towards the ceiling and then extending it.
- Return the dumbbell to the start position in a controlled manner.

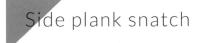

Side plank with leg raise

- Set up in a regular side plank.
- Raise and lower your upper leg while maintaining the plank position.

Both of these movements can either be performed for time, targeting 60 seconds, or, especially for the side plank snatch, you can work to reps (i.e. 3 x 10) with a higher load.

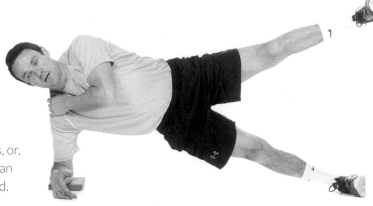

Group exercise classes and CrossFit

Whether it's an informal circuit session organised in the off season by your cycling club, a military-boot-camp-style class or CrossFit, group exercise sessions can be a fun and motivating option for off the bike training. There's no doubt that these types of classes get a lot of people exercising who might not if they were on their own, but should they be part of your regular training routine?

There are a number of factors to bear in mind when considering taking part in a class and, if you do decide to participate, ways you can minimise your risk of injury and maximise the gains you'll get.

It's important to be aware of the distinction between exercise and training. Exercise is physical activity for its possible health benefits. Training is physical activity with a longer-term goal in mind, usually improved performance in a particular sport. The nature of group classes is that they tend to fit into the first category and, as such, tend to be fairly random in nature with regard to the exercises and movements prescribed. You'll probably end up doing some exercises that may benefit your cycling but it's likely to be more through luck than planning. Also, if there are 30 participants in a class all doing the same exercise, you can almost guarantee that it won't be suitable for them all. One of the premises of this book is that a one-size-fits-all approach is far from ideal for off the bike conditioning and, unfortunately, the very nature of group classes means they fall into this camp.

In theory, all exercises can be modified or scaled to the participants, but in a group environment it's unlikely that the instructor will be able to make the personalised coaching interventions to ensure correct form across the whole class. Many such classes are businesses and, as such, more participants mean more money for the instructor or gym. It's also important to remember that their technical training may be fairly limited, especially when dealing with any injury concerns. Also, the ethos of many of these classes is to keep pushing and this can cause individuals to go dangerously beyond their physical capabilities. Obviously pushing beyond your perceived limitations can be a good thing as

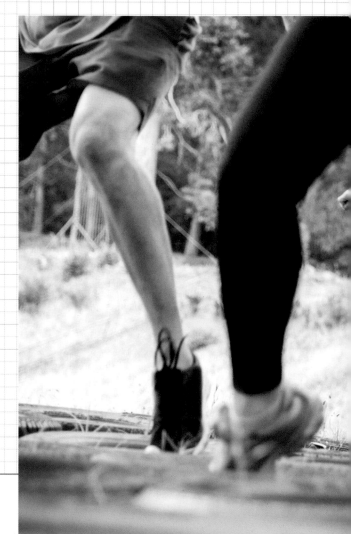

it's one of the premises for improvement, adaptation and increasing your capacity for work. However, it's important to be mindful of any injury risks and the potential issues of overtraining.

There's no doubt that if you follow the assessment and exercise recommendations in this book, your body will be far more suited and able to cope with the demands of this style of workout. You'll also be more aware of your current limitations and be able to make more informed judgements as to whether a particular exercise is suitable for you.

We're definitely not saying that you should steer clear of group classes, but it's essential that you approach them in a mindful and body-aware manner. If an exercise doesn't feel right or you sense that your form is starting to fail, make a modification, stop or skip it. Don't feel pressured by the instructor, the atmosphere of the class or your own ego – your main goal is riding strong, not being the best in a circuit class!

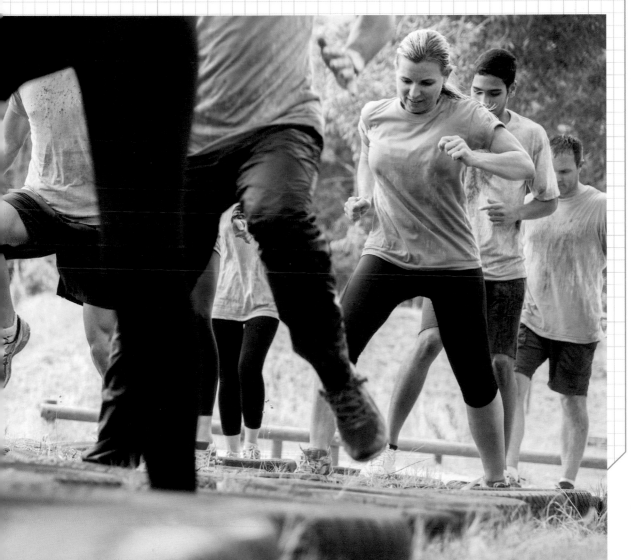

▼ *Exercising in a group can be motivating but don't be afraid to say no if an exercise doesn't feel right to you.*

Machines versus free weights

Whenever people talk about resistance training, there are debates about whether one mode of training is better than another. One of the more common debates is around whether to perform free weight exercises, such as those in this book, or machine-based exercises.

There are arguments for and against each mode of training. However, there are benefits to be had from performing both types of resistance training. Many people sit in one camp or the other when it comes to machines or free weights. We don't really see why it has to be an either/or case.

Making the choice as to which modality to use comes down, as with most things, to what you want to achieve. Once you know what you are trying to achieve, you find the right tools for the purpose. You wouldn't use a screwdriver to hammer in nails and, in the same way, for some training goals machines are more applicable, while for others free weights are the preferred option.

In the case of machines, we have used machine weight-training activities for specific reasons with elite athletes for a number of different purposes:

1 When an athlete is injured or is returning from an injury, machine-based weight training can be a useful modality to have a training effect without stressing the injured part (for example, the use of a unilateral leg press when an athlete has an injury in the other leg).

2 When an athlete needs to develop a certain muscle group or action. For example, if an athlete has a quad/hamstring ratio that is causing knee issues, there may be a need to programme specific hamstring work. Machines are a useful way to overload a muscle group.

However, machines also have their limitations, the key one being that they operate in fixed planes of movement. At the start of this book, we talked about cycling being a 'narrow' activity, so in this case we actually want to get away from fixed ranges of movement and challenge the body outside of one plane, to develop that wide conditioning base. That is why, in this book, the exercises are primarily free exercises to challenge the body in three dimensions, which forces many of the smaller muscles that get neglected or underused in cycling activity to work and improve the health and well-being of the body.

◄ *Fixed weight machines have a place in some training scenarios but, in general, free weight exercises are preferable.*

Plan to succeed
Once you're at this stage of the programme, planning your year, weeks, days and individual sessions correctly is essential. Determine the demands of your chosen target events and the times of year when strength work is most appropriate. By planning well, you will minimise any negative interference between your strength work and cycling training, and maximise the gains you'll achieve.

Taper into events
Part of this planning is tapering down to important events and this applies equally to both your off the bike training and your on the bike work. It shouldn't be a sudden stop but a planned and progressive winding down. All athletes respond differently to tapering, so although we have given guidelines, you may need to experiment and adapt to find what's optimal for you.

Don't forget the basics
Just because you've reached this stage of the programme, don't think you're done with the assessment and corrective exercises. Still try to work daily on the TASMT and stretching exercises that you know apply to you and regularly work through the assessment to check you're still fit to lift. For the majority of riders, progressing with loading and developing the exercises in Chapter 4 will provide a long-term challenge, so don't rush trying to include the more advanced exercises or set/rep structures.

Schedule your strength sessions
Within your training week, schedule your strength work to allow a minimum of 48 hours between sessions and aim for minimal interference with your cycling. If you find that this is not the case, revisit your overall plan and maybe change the priority of the training block.

Prioritise your weaknesses
In each strength session, you should be looking to include a hinge, a squat/split squat, a push, a pull and ideally a trunk movement. You should work on the movement you find most difficult or challenging first, when you're fresher both mentally and physically. It's quite likely that you won't be at the same level for all movements and, for example, although you may be on Chapter 5 exercises for your upper body, you may still be patterning and cementing for the lower body movements. This will constantly change, which is the reason that regularly revisiting the assessment is so vital.

CHAPTER SUMMARY

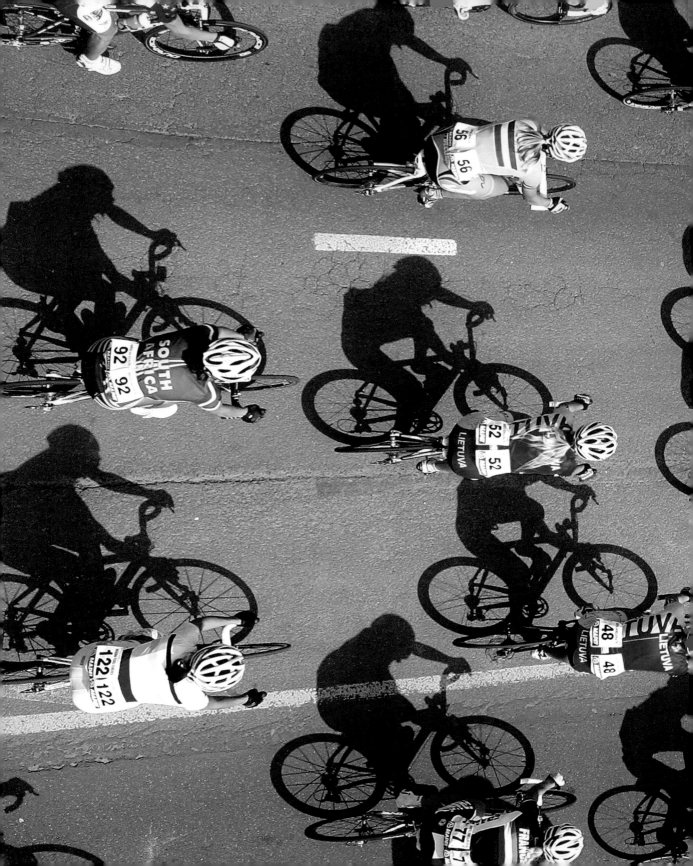

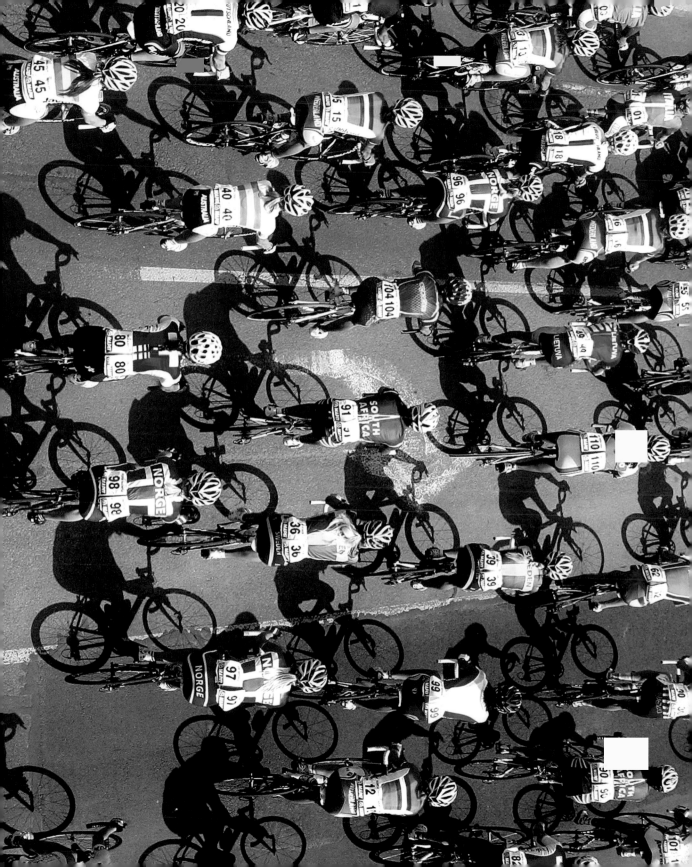

REFERENCES AND FURTHER READING

REFERENCES

Mujika et al., 2016
https://www.researchgate.net/publication/301274212_
Effects_of_Increased_Muscle_Strength_and_Muscle_
Mass_on_Endurance-Cycling_Performance

Ronnestad et al., 2010
https://www.researchgate.net/publication/46010265_
In-season_strength_maintenance_training_increases_
well-trained_cyclists%27_performance

Ronnestad et al. 2011
https://www.ncbi.nlm.nih.gov/pubmed/19903319

Ronnestad et al. 2015
https://www.researchgate.net/publication/275102845_
Strength_training_improves_cycling_performance_
fractional_utilization_of_VO2max_and_cycling_
economy_in_female_cyclists

FURTHER READING

https://www.researchgate.net/publication/305802930_
10_weeks_of_heavy_strength_training_improves_
performance-related_measurements_in_elite_cyclists

https://www.researchgate.net/publication/315056975_
Heavy_strength_training_improves_running_and_cycling_
performance_following_prolonged_submaximal_work_
in_well-trained_female_athletes

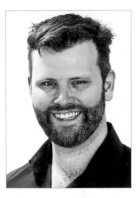

Phil Burt qualified as a physiotherapist in 1999 and since then has worked with some of the best athletes in the world across a number of sports. In 2006 he started to work with British Cycling and through his dynamic, world leading approach quickly became the lead physiotherapist to the teams that dominated cycling at the 2008 Beijing, 2012 London and 2016 Rio Games. He was an active member of the 'Secret Squirrel club' and was the driving innovative force behind a number of projects benefitting both performance and rider health. His work on saddle issues led to the UCI changing their ruling on saddle angle. He is a world authority on bike fit and is on the Rëtul World Board of Advisors and the Cyclefit Symposium organising committee. He consults for other elite organisations including the SAS and English Premier League Football. His previous book, *Bike Fit: Optimise your bike position for high performance and injury avoidance*, has been a top seller and has helped countless riders to more comfortable, successful and injury free cycling. Having left British Cycling in 2018, he has set-up philburtinnovation.co.uk . He offers a range of services including cycling specific injury assessment and treatment, bike fit, aero appraisals and saddle health checks. He's also makes bespoke product solutions and innovations to make cycling more comfortable for everyone. An internationally renowned public speaker-he aims to ride his bike everyday he can.

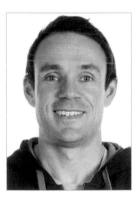

Martin Evans graduated with a 1st Class BSc in Sports and Exercise Science in 2003 and followed this with a Post Graduate Diploma with Distinction in Coaching Science. He was a senior strength & conditioning coach at the English Institute of Sport (EIS), working as the Lead Strength & Conditioning Coach for British Cycling. Working across the Great Britain Cycling Team with endurance riders and sprinters alike, his role was pivotal to both performance on the bike and injury avoidance off it. The strength and conditioning strategy that he developed was used to support all athletes on the Great Britain Cycling Team programme. He was a crucial member of the team that prepared the athletes for their world beating performances at the London 2012 and Rio 2016 Olympics & Paralympics. He is now the Women's Physical Performance Lead at the Football Association and oversees the physical preparation strategy for all of the Women's International Teams. He has also worked as part of a multi-disciplinary sports science and medical team at the EIS. His experience also spans across a range of sports including swimming, triathlon and rugby at an international level.

INDEX

Assessment flow diagram

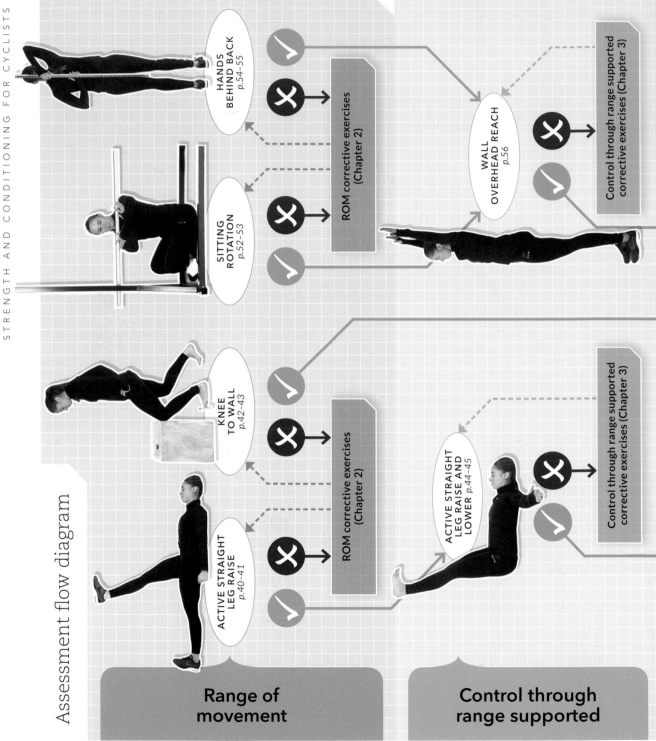

Range of movement

ACTIVE STRAIGHT LEG RAISE *p.40–41*

KNEE TO WALL *p.42–43*

SITTING ROTATION *p.52–53*

HANDS BEHIND BACK *p.54–55*

ROM corrective exercises (Chapter 2)

Control through range supported

ACTIVE STRAIGHT LEG RAISE AND LOWER *p.44–45*

WALL OVERHEAD REACH *p.56*

Control through range supported corrective exercises (Chapter 3)

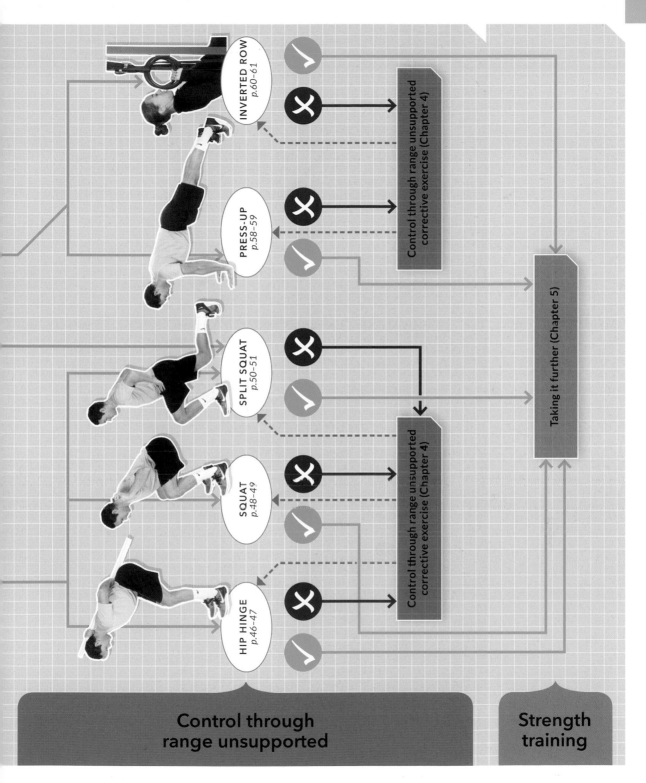

INVERTED ROW
p.60–61

PRESS-UP
p.58–59

SPLIT SQUAT
p.50–51

SQUAT
p.48–49

HIP HINGE
p.46–47

Control through range unsupported corrective exercise (Chapter 4)

Control through range unsupported corrective exercise (Chapter 4)

Taking it further (Chapter 5)

Control through range unsupported

Strength training

ACKNOWLEDGEMENTS

We would like to thank those who helped make this book possible: Nik Cook, Charlotte Croft, Sarah Skipper, David Luxton and Ruth Waghorn. Without your support and guidance it is unlikely we would have got to this point.

We would also like to thank our families: Phil's wife Claire, and children Noah and Esme and Martin's girlfriend, Kath, whose combined patience allowed us the time to write.

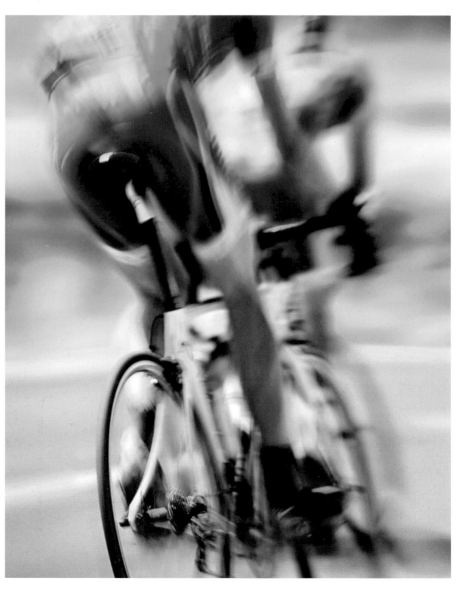